Applied Demography Series

Series Editor
David A.Swanson

More information about this series at http://www.springer.com/series/8838

Richard K. Thomas

In Sickness and In Health

Disease and Disability in Contemporary America

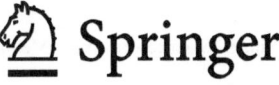 Springer

Richard K. Thomas
MEMPHIS, TN, US

ISSN 2352-376X   ISSN 2352-3778   (electronic)
Applied Demography Series
ISBN 978-1-4939-3421-8   ISBN 978-1-4939-3423-2   (eBook)
DOI 10.1007/978-1-4939-3423-2

Library of Congress Control Number: 2015954393

Springer New York Heidelberg Dordrecht London

Printed on acid-free paper

Springer Science+Business Media LLC New York is part of Springer Science+Business Media
(www.springer.com)

Preface

The study of morbidity has become a growing focus of demographers for a number of reasons. These include the growing emphasis on population health, the declining significance of mortality, and the shift from an emphasis on acute conditions to chronic conditions, among other developments. The interest in morbidity on the part of demographers, epidemiologists, health planners, and medical scientists steadily increased over the last quarter of the twentieth century as the connection between demographic variables and morbidity differentials became clearer. Although perhaps still lagging behind more traditional spheres of demographic inquiry, the literature available on morbidity has grown and findings from research in this field are driving much of the current thought in healthcare. It is increasingly understood that many advances in our understanding and management of the contemporary health problems reflect a better understanding of the demographic dimensions of morbidity.

This interest in morbidity has developed against a backdrop of increasing demand for health-related data of all types. A diverse set of entities that historically had little interest in or need for health-related data now realize that efficient data gathering and analysis are necessary for carrying out their respective functions. Today's healthcare environment is demanding improvements in the quality, quantity, and specificity of the data used for research, marketing, planning, and business development.

Epidemiologists have expanded our understanding of the relationship between disease incidence and demographic factors. Indeed, the persistent health disparities correlated with demographic attributes have become a major focus of research. Population scientists have increasingly recognized the importance of the study of morbidity rather than mortality as a measure of the health of society. Policy makers grappling with societal-level issues like Medicare's future viability or simply addressing basic healthcare needs at the local level are increasingly relying on morbidity data as a basis for decision making. Healthcare organizations striving to adapt to a rapidly changing environment must understand trends in morbidity for purposes of survival. The passage of the Patient Protection and Affordable Care Act in 2010 served to further underscore the importance of such information.

The demand for morbidity data, in fact, has grown far beyond the organizations directly involved in the provision of healthcare. Health plans, employers, policy makers, health lawyers, and a variety of other interests increasingly require such data. Entities both inside and outside of healthcare are now using morbidity data not only for understanding disease patterns but also for planning, marketing, and business development, as well as for cost containment, quality monitoring, and legal purposes. Entire issues of scholarly journals have been devoted to debates regarding the management of information for these purposes, and as the population health movement gains momentum, additional resources are likely to be added to this body of knowledge.

Access to quality morbidity data is required not only for those involved in health services research, planning, and evaluation but also for the effective operation of the healthcare system. On a basic level, accurate morbidity data are required for disease tracking and for the implementation of disease management programs. The shift in the burden of disease from acute conditions to chronic conditions has amplified the needs for (and gaps in) critical data. Morbidity data are required for determining the needs for health services, facilities, and personnel. Any planning activities in the healthcare arena rely heavily on incidence and prevalence data for various health conditions. Efforts to evaluate the effectiveness of health interventions rely on the availability of morbidity data. Additionally, recent research highlights significant small-area variability in morbidity patterns indicating the need for high-quality morbidity data at the community level.

While the demand for morbidity data has grown as a result of various trends in healthcare, the availability of quality data has not kept pace. This lack of data, coupled with issues of data quality, accessibility, and usefulness, represents a challenge for health professionals, researchers, and demographers. The increase in demand for morbidity data has exposed the weaknesses in the availability and accessibility of comprehensive and timely data on disease prevalence and disability. This is particularly the case for information on the "true" prevalence of health problems within a population and information on the "known cases" within a population. Since there is no central repository of data on the amount and distribution of health conditions or the use of services within a population, it is impossible to generate actual data on morbidity. The fact that data on hospital admissions are available in some locales but not others allows only a partial view of the level of sickness and disability within the population.

This situation demands a comprehensive review of the state of the art with regard to morbidity data. This book is intended to survey the current state of morbidity data in the US, describe its characteristics and availability, and provide guidance to those who require morbidity data for the variety of uses to which such information might be put. This practical knowledge is supplemented by material that addresses changes in morbidity patterns and their implications for demographic processes and social change. This book does not represent an end to the discussion of morbidity but a beginning as efforts are undertaken to improve the availability, accessibility, and usefulness of data on sickness and disability.

Richard K. Thomas

Contents

Chapter 1
Introduction to the Study of Morbidity

Morbidity , in its simplest terms, refers to the level of sickness and disability exhibited by a population. The term "morbidity" comes from the Latin "morbus" for disease and "morbidus" for diseased. Morbidity has been of interest to human societies throughout history as people have struggled to understand sickness and death. Social commentators have long recorded the impact of disease on human populations, and the precursors of the modern medical scientists were faced with the responsibility for explaining and managing the sickness characteristic of their respective societies.

Demographers have traditionally focused on the study of mortality (the end result of morbidity), and only in recent years has the emphasis shifted more in the direction of morbidity. As morbidity has come to be more reflective of the nature of a society's health problems than mortality, the interest in the study of morbidity has increased. The current concern over disparities in health status—disparities most often described in demographic terms—has attracted increased attention to what demography can bring to this discussion, and the study of morbidity, of course, is a key component of health demography.

While "morbidity" may be used to refer to the health status of an individual or a group, demographers are almost exclusively interested in morbidity as associated with populations and rarely with the morbidity of individuals. It is, after all, the health status of populations and subpopulations that is of interest to health demographers. The exception to this might be the situation in which the identified health status of individuals based on some assessment tool is aggregated to generate the morbidity status of the population in question.

A number of factors have contributed to the growing significance accorded to morbidity by representatives of a variety of disciplines. These include:

The declining significance of mortality. The study of mortality is one of the three principal areas of focus for demographers, and early students of epidemiology focused on mortality and its causes in their efforts to understand the impact of disease and injury on the health of the population. During the twentieth century, the mortality

© Springer New York 2016
R.K. Thomas, *In Sickness and In Health*, Applied Demography Series 6,
DOI 10.1007/978-1-4939-3423-2_1

rate fell dramatically, resulting in not only fewer deaths proportionately within the population but also a less significant role for mortality in population change.

The shift in emphasis from acute conditions to chronic conditions. At the same time that the impact of mortality on the population was declining, the major causes of death were shifting from acute conditions (principally communicable diseases) to chronic conditions. This "epidemiologic transition" served to increase the interest in the study of diseases and their distribution within the population. At the same time, the complex etiology and course of chronic diseases created a challenge for medical researchers and population scientists. While acute conditions affect a cross section of the population seemingly at random, chronic diseases are much more selective in their impact resulting in demographically related disparities in health status.

Growth of lifestyle-generated conditions. The preponderance of health problems confronting Americans today are "diseases of civilization," conditions that reflect the lifestyles characterizing contemporary US society. In fact, some 80 % of deaths are now attributed to lifestyle-related conditions. This phenomenon is of particular interest to demographers since differential lifestyles are typically associated with various demographic groups within society. Some demographic segments are more likely to use alcohol and drugs or exhibit unsafe sexual practices than others. Some segments are more likely to follow healthy diets and get adequate exercise than others. In fact, complex classification systems have been developed that link demographic traits to various lifestyle categories.

Persistent disparities in health status. Medical practitioners and policy makers are increasingly concerned over the disparities that continue to exist in health status among various segments of the population. Morbidity levels for some demographic segments are persistently higher than those in other segments. Being African-American or Hispanic, for example, means higher rates of both acute and chronic conditions, higher acuity of conditions, and more negative clinical outcomes. These disparities can also be found related to income, educational level, and other factors and can only be addressed through an in-depth understanding of the demographic correlates of health and illness.

The impact of newly emerging and re-emerging diseases. In recent years, the interest in morbidity has grown due to evidence that certain new diseases have emerged within the US population (either through external introduction or the development of antibiotic-resistant strains of existing diseases). At the same time, certain diseases long thought eradicated in the US have begun to resurface, prompting renewed interest in the study of disease etiology and distribution. Current patterns of immigration have opened the doors for the introduction (or reintroduction) of certain communicable diseases.

Public interest in contributions to good health. By the last third of the twentieth century, the population of the US (and other developed countries) had developed an interest (even an obsession) with healthy living. Americans have increasingly accessed the growing body of information that documents the effect of various diets and health practices on their quality of life. The interest in the prevention and management of various conditions on the part of consumers has served to increase the demand for information on the factors that contribute to health status even among both health professionals and the general public.

The recurrent issue of healthcare reform. Observers have long noted the range of problems that are associated with the US healthcare system. There are problems related to access, equity, quality, cost, and a variety of other factors. As the public discussion of healthcare issues has increased, the spotlight has shown more clearly on deficiencies in the healthcare system that impact morbidity. Debate surrounding reform of the health insurance industry, the solvency of the Medicare program, and the future of medical education, for example, must be informed by an understanding of the morbidity patterns of the US population. These morbidity characteristics had more than a little influence on the enactment of the Patient Protection and Affordable Care Act of 2010.

The growing interest in "population health." There is growing interest in the concept of "population health" among health professionals, policy analysts, and government agencies. Given the obvious deficiencies of the US healthcare system, a more "wholesale" approach that addresses the healthcare needs of groups of people—rather than individual patients—seems to be increasingly inevitable. New approaches to addressing the health problems of the US population are needed, and not-for-profit hospitals must now demonstrate that they are addressing the healthcare needs of the total service area population and not just their patients. This effort involves the identification of and attention to the non-medical factors that influence health status and the social contributors to ill-health, factors clearly addressed through demographically oriented morbidity analyses.

The growing emphasis on evaluation and outcomes measures. Government agencies, regulators, insurance plans, and health policy analysts are increasingly interested in the outcomes generated by health improvement efforts at the clinical (individual) level and the health status (population) level. Providers are being asked to demonstrate that their efforts are producing outcomes that meet certain standards, and pay-for-performance is becoming increasingly common. In order to demonstrate the impact of the provision of health services for individuals or populations, health professionals require access to comprehensive, timely, and detailed data on the morbidity levels of the populations for which they have responsibility.

Who Studies Morbidity?

Although morbidity has not historically been one of the most studied topics by demographers, the interest in morbidity analysis has increased concomitant to the growing appreciation of the demographic correlates of health status and health behavior. The fact that the distribution of morbidity within the US population mirrors the distribution of demographic characteristics has spurred the development of the field of health demography. From an applied demography perspective, efforts toward addressing issues in healthcare today can be informed through an understanding of the interface between demography and health-related characteristics.

Epidemiologists have historically studied the morbidity patterns characterizing populations. Whether as medical doctors specializing in epidemiology or public health officials, epidemiologists represent the first line of interface with morbid events within the population. While the work of health demographers is informed by epidemiology, epidemiologists today can benefit from the growing body of research linking demographic traits to patterns of morbidity.

Public health officials have a particular interest in morbidity patterns, although from a different perspective than clinicians. With their emphasis on population health, public health officials focus on broad patterns of disease within the population and examine the association between disease incidence and the population's demographic attributes. Efforts by public health officials to reduce morbidity begin with an understanding of the demographic characteristics of the target population.

Healthcare administrators must organize their services to meet the needs of the populations they serve, and these services should reflect the morbidity patterns of that population. Today's professional administrators recognize the need to match services offered with the health services needs of the population. This requires that the service area population be carefully profiled in terms of its demographic characteristics and that these characteristics be converted into demand estimates that determine the type and number of services required.

Health insurance plans require information on the morbidity characteristics of those enrolled in their plans or those parties they intend to market to. The rationale behind health insurance is that the insurer can "bet" that their plan members will pay in more premiums than the insurance company has to pay out in claims. For existing covered lives, health insurance companies typically have detailed internal information on the morbidity experiences of their plan members. For prospective enrollees, it is incumbent upon them to develop prospective morbidity profiles. Their ability to win the bet rests on their understanding of the morbidity risks associated with their plan members.

Health planners work in a variety of settings that include government agencies, public health departments, health systems, and consumer health products companies. Regardless of the planning activity undertaken, health planners are particularly interested in the demographic characteristics of the population under study and, subsequently, in the morbidity profile of that population. The importance of health planning, long neglected, is being ratcheted up due to, among other developments, requirements pursuant to the Affordable Care Act of 2010. Thus, there will be a need to profile the characteristics of potential participants in state- or federally run insurance exchanges, examine the characteristics of the additional people who will be eligible to participate in Medicaid, and conduct mandated community health needs assessments for not-for-profit hospitals.

A wide variety of healthcare entities, whether providers of care, producers of medical supplies and drugs, or organizations providing goods or services to the healthcare industry, are required to market themselves to their prospective customers. Healthcare marketing has become increasingly data driven and this has increased the need for a wide range of health-related data, including morbidity data. The ability to profile a target audience in terms of its morbidity characteristics and its health service needs is becoming increasingly critical for successful marketing initiatives.

One final group with an interest in morbidity is health policy analysts and policy makers. Given the impact on the US economy on activities within the healthcare arena there is significant and growing interest in the factors that contribute to the increasing cost of meeting the healthcare needs of the US population. Government policy analysts responsible for programs such as Medicare, Medicaid, and Social Security have an urgent need for comprehensive, timely, and detailed data on American morbidity patterns. Such information is used to inform policy decisions with regard to issues as basic as reimbursement rates for physicians under Medicare to issues as broad as eligibility for the Medicaid program.

Why Do They Study It?

The most basic reason for studying morbidity and morbidity patterns is to develop an understanding of the amount and nature of sickness and disability within the US population. The basic questions include: (1) what sicknesses exist within US society? (2) what is the incidence/prevalence of the conditions?: and (3) what is the distribution of these conditions in both geographic and demographic terms? This baseline information can be expanded by determining who gets sick and what they get sick from. It is clear that morbid conditions are not randomly distributed within the population but are concentrated within certain segments of it. It has been suggested that 20 % of the population accounts for 80 % of the health problems. This being the case, it is important to identify the segments of the population that are most likely to be affected by various health conditions.

Morbidity has become an increasingly important topic of study for demographers, partly because trends in morbidity patterns are becoming increasingly significant in explaining the population's health status, its patterns of mortality, and even its changing population characteristics. The distribution of morbidity within modern populations is highly correlated with demographic variables. Age, sex, and race are important predictors of morbidity, with income, educational attainment, employment status, and even religious affiliation being correlated with health status.

These studies can be taken even further with an examination of the causes of differentials seen in the distribution and level of morbid conditions within a population. What factors lead to the emergence of various diseases and explain their distribution within the population? Why are some groups more susceptible to certain health conditions than others? What factors might trigger the onset of health conditions in some populations but not others? This analysis can be extended further to examine the impact of demographic traits on the progression of disease, disease prognoses, and ultimate disposition of the affected individuals.

While the development of a baseline understanding of morbidity is important, ultimately the challenge is to apply this information to concrete problems in the real world. Applied demographers, population scientists, epidemiologists, and others use this information to plan public health initiatives, develop treatment modalities, improve the delivery of care, and develop marketing programs for healthcare organizations.

In order to address the pressing challenges of the day, morbidity data can be utilized to better manage chronic conditions, for the development of effective health insurance plans (private and public), to address the financial challenges facing Medicare, and a myriad of other challenges within the healthcare area.

Intrinsic in the application of morbidity data to health issues is the need to allocate scarce resources. Public health agencies have long been financially constrained and forced to make hard decisions with regard to resource allocation. In today's environment, even for-profit healthcare organizations are faced with the need to maximize resources, and this means having the information necessary to make rational allocation decisions. Public health agencies have to determine where the expenditure of resources will provide the most public health bang for the buck, not-for-profit healthcare entities must develop cost-effective approaches to the provision of care, and for-profit healthcare entities may be involved in marketing activities that require an understanding of the population segments with the greatest potential as customers. Research institutes must determine which conditions merit the expenditure of resources and which are of secondary importance.

The Interrelationship Between Demography and Morbidity

The morbidity characteristics of a population are related directly and indirectly to the demographic structure of that population. On the one hand, the demographic makeup of the population is a key determinant of the type of health problems exhibited by that population. On the other hand, the morbidity profile of a population influences the demographic structure of that population. In addition, the key demographic processes characterizing a population (i.e., fertility, mortality, and migration) each influence the morbidity patterns of the population, while that population's morbidity patterns concurrently influence its morbidity processes.

A population's demographic makeup is a critical determinant of its morbidity characteristics. For the US population today, factors such as age distribution, sex ratio, racial and ethnic makeup, and even attributes such as marital status, income, and education influence the extant types of health problems. An overriding issue in America today is the changing age distribution and its implications for morbidity. As the US population has aged it has undergone an epidemiological transition in which chronic conditions have replaced acute conditions as the predominant health problems and most frequent causes of death. The aging of the population has resulted in a growing "excess" of women thereby affecting the configuration of the morbidity profile. Increasing racial and ethnic diversity (not to mention unprecedented levels of immigration) has had an impact on morbidity patterns and even such factors as changing household structures and occupational patterns influence the morbidity picture.

Similarly, the morbidity profile of the population has implications for its demographic makeup. Sickness (and subsequent death rates) has a significant impact on population size and composition. A reduction in infant and childhood diseases (and the potential for infant and child mortality) has been a major contributor to increased life expectancy. Higher morbidity rates for some segments of the population result in higher levels of disability which in turn impact the educational and economic potential of these populations. Preventable deaths at an early age ultimately modify the demographic profile of these populations.

The major demographic processes also interact with a population's other attributes to influence morbidity patterns. Differential fertility patterns, for example, contribute directly and indirectly to the observed morbidity profile. High fertility rates among low-income and poorly educated segments of the population contribute to higher levels of infant and child morbidity and ultimately to infant mortality rates that are higher than those of comparable countries. Births to very young women and very old women are considered high risk and, to the extent they account for a significant proportion of the births, affect the incidence of various health conditions. At the same time, the declining mortality rate has interacted with the epidemiological transition to influence the contemporary morbidity profile.

The fact that more people are living longer has resulted in an increase in the proportion of the population with a chronic condition, and large numbers of elderly mean that an unprecedented proportion of the population is characterized by multiple chronic conditions. Three or four generations ago, few people lived long enough to contract the chronic conditions that are common today, with the aging of the population serving to reduce the significance of acute conditions. The high rate of immigration over the past 20 years has changed not only the demographic makeup of the US population but also its morbidity profile. First generation immigrants are by and large healthier than native-born Americans, although they are more likely to be affected by certain communicable and infectious diseases that are rare within the US population or have been previously eradicated. Subsequently, the health status of second- and third-generation immigrants tends to decline, adopting a health status profile similar to that of native-born Americans.

Evidence of the Growing Importance of Morbidity Analysis

The interest in morbidity on the part of demographers, epidemiologists, health planners, and medical scientists steadily increased during the late twentieth century. The body of research on this topic has expanded dramatically although perhaps still lagging behind more traditional spheres of demographic analysis. The literature available on morbidity has grown, and findings from research in this field are driving much of the current thought in healthcare. Some of the evidence for the growing significance of morbidity analysis is presented below.

Emergence of health demography as a distinct field. During the 1980s a separate field in demography devoted to the study of the relationship between demography and various aspects of health and healthcare began to emerge. While the fledgling field of health demography encompassed all aspects of demographic analysis as related to healthcare, much of the focus was on morbidity. Sessions devoted to health demography or this topic under some other name increased at the professional meetings of a variety of disciplines. The emergence of health demography and its basic tenets were summarized in the work of Pol and Thomas (2013).

The shift in the focus of research funding. Research funding in the US has historically been devoted to efforts to treat and cure acute conditions. Originating during the heyday of the medical model of care, research understandably focused on the pressing healthcare threats of the day. It was not until the epidemiologic transition was well underway that the research emphasis began to shift from a focus on acute conditions to a focus on chronic conditions. Once underway, it became clear that understanding chronic disease and its management represented a much greater challenge than did acute conditions. The complexity of chronic disease etiology, its sometimes unpredictable progression, and its management challenges presented issues not previously faced by researchers. More attention began to be paid to disease etiology, the progression of disease, and case management with an emphasis on the demographic disparities associated with chronic disease.

The paradigm shift from medical care to healthcare. Probably the most significant development in healthcare during the last quarter of the twentieth century was the shift that occurred from an emphasis on "medical care" to one on "healthcare." While it is difficult to determine which came first—the emergence of a new paradigm focusing on a more broadly defined healthcare model driven by chronic diseases or the growing body of research on chronic disease that contributed to the rise of the healthcare model—this paradigm shift was accompanied by a growing interest in the study of morbidity. While acute conditions generally affect a cross section of the population without respect to age, sex, or race, chronic conditions are much more selective in their impact. Implicit in the development of the new healthcare model was an appreciation for the demographic correlates of disease onset, disease progression, and disease outcomes.

Increasing demand for morbidity data. Virtually every development in healthcare whether it relates to personal health or national healthcare policy setting is driving the need for better morbidity data. Increasing competition between healthcare providers for patients and among health insurers for plan members, the requirements instituted under the 2010 Affordable Care Act, deliberations on the future of Medicare, and many other developments require an understanding of the characteristics of patients, their health status, and their health behavior. Healthcare as an industry has become increasingly data driven and the demand for more complete, detailed, and timely morbidity can be expected to extend well into the future.

Audience for the Book

This book was initially envisioned as a step toward filling a void in the demographic literature. It was subsequently chosen for inclusion in the Springer series on applied demography. Demographers represent the immediate audience for this work, particularly those involved in applied demography and health demography. Public health officials, epidemiologists, and biostatisticians all require ever higher "doses" of morbidity data. At the same time, a growing number of health professionals require access to morbidity data for clinical decision-making, administrative policy setting, and health services research. Students in demography, public health, health services research, and even healthcare administration should find this book useful, along with practitioners and consultants in those fields. Health professionals in both the public and private sectors involved in health services planning, administration, or evaluation should also benefit from this book.

The book can serve as both a reference work and a classroom text. Virtually everyone in healthcare must be familiar with these concepts in today's environment, regardless of the aspect of healthcare with which they deal. The glossary provided should be useful to a wide range of individuals.

Organization of the Book

The book is organized in such a manner as to achieve the following objectives:

1. To define morbidity and related terms
2. To provide an overview of morbidity data in its various forms
3. To document the substantial and growing need for morbidity data of all types
4. To summarize the various categories of morbidity data, the ways in which these data are generated, and the means of accessing these data
5. To provide guidance in assessing the quality, accessibility, and usefulness of these sources
6. To demonstrate the availability of morbidity data at various levels of geography
7. To describe methods for synthetically generating morbidity data
8. To suggest future opportunities for the generation and dissemination of morbidity data

Chapter 1 has presented an introduction to the study of morbidity, discussed the various dimensions of the field, traced the history of the study of morbidity, and identified those who study morbidity and why they study it. Chapter 2 expands on the definitions of key concepts presented in Chap. 1, including such critical concepts as health, sickness, disease, and disability among others, and describes their relevance for the study of morbidity. Chapter 3 provides an overview of the ways in which morbidity data can be categorized, the ways different parties view and utilize the data, and the various official classification systems that are used in healthcare and other arenas.

After the presentation of the basics of the study of morbidity, Chap. 4 examines issues involved in the identification (i.e., case finding) of morbidity within a population and the methods available for quantifying the amount of morbidity. The various measures utilized are reviewed and efforts to develop health status indicators discussed. Chapter 5 addresses the issue of measuring morbidity within a population and comes to grips with the issue of determining how sick a population is. Chapters 6 and 7 examine the factors that influence morbidity, including demographic correlates, lifestyle patterns, environmental considerations, and structural factors (e.g., access to healthcare). These chapters lay the groundwork for Chap. 8 which reviews the current state of morbidity in the US, traces changes in the patterns of morbidity over the past century, and discusses the implications of changing morbidity patterns for both healthcare and society in general. Chapter 9 describes the available sources of morbidity data and identifies the entities that generate morbidity data, along with the mechanisms for disseminating this information. This final chapter provides an assessment of available data options, ways to evaluate the various sources, and guidance in determing the best source for a particular application.

Following the chapters, an extensive glossary of terms and concepts related to morbidity and associated topics is provided, including "official" terminology used by government agencies and technical terms from the healthcare field.

Reference

Pol, L., & Thomas, R. K. (2013). *The demography of health and healthcare* (3rd ed.). New York: Springer.

Chapter 2
Basic Concepts in Morbidity Analysis

A number of concepts must be understood in order to examine the nature of sickness and disability within the US population. Some of these concepts are drawn from medical science while others have social science roots. Many are precisely defined while others are more subjective and characterized by amorphous definitions that may be situational in nature. The key concepts and terms useful for morbidity analysis are discussed below.

Morbidity

Morbidity refers to the level of sickness and disability characterizing a population. The term "morbidity" (and its root "morbid") is derived from the Latin "morbus" for disease and "morbidus" for diseased. While the term has specific meaning for epidemiologists, "morbidity" and related terms may be used in various ways inside and outside of the scientific community. Thus, one hears reference to a "morbid curiosity" or the "morbid details," and other terms that may not reflect the scientific meaning of the word.

Morbidity has been of interest to human societies throughout history as people have struggled to understand sickness and death. Demographers traditionally focused on the study of mortality (the end result of morbidity), and only in recent years has the emphasis shifted more in the direction of morbidity. As morbidity has come to play a greater role in shaping the nature of society than mortality, the interest in this topic has increased. Indeed, the current concern over disparities in health status—disparities most often described in demographic terms—has attracted increased attention to the perspective that demographers can bring to this discussion.

© Springer New York 2016
R.K. Thomas, *In Sickness and In Health*, Applied Demography Series 6,
DOI 10.1007/978-1-4939-3423-2_2

For our purposes, morbidity refers to the state of being ill, diseased or disabled. While most scholars would concur with this working definition, it does raise the question of what constitutes being ill or diseased. Does this mean that a condition has been "officially" diagnosed by a medical practitioner? Does the condition have to alter health status or affect one's quality of life before it is counted? Is a physical disability really a disability if it doesn't interfere with one's activities? Ultimately, the application of the definition depends on the assumptions made by those evaluating the health of the population and the standards established by society.

Morbidity may be used to refer to a person or a group, with the former referring to the health status of an individual and the latter to the health status of a population. Demographers are, of course, almost exclusively interested in morbidity as associated with populations and seldom with the morbidity of individuals, thus the distinction between individual (clinical) morbidity and group (epidemiological) morbidity. The exception to this might be the situation in which the identified health status of individuals is available but population-level data are not.

This distinction raises the question of whether group morbidity is the sum of individual morbidity or, rather, population-based morbidity is qualitatively different from cumulative individual morbidity. Those coming at the issue from a clinical perspective are more likely to support the former representation, while those emphasizing a population health approach are likely to opt for the latter. A good case could be made that societal morbidity is more than the sum of its constituent parts. In fact, it could be argued that in communities that exhibit persistently poor health status, something of a "subculture of ill-health" emerges that fosters rather than inhibits poor health. This perspective would contend that health problems cannot be understood at the individual level (i.e., one patient at a time) and that a holistic approach is required that takes into consideration not only the affected individuals but also the environments that contribute to morbidity.

The morbidity level within a population can be quantified in a number of ways and these will be discussed in detail in Chap. 3. For our purposes here, we should note that distinctions can be made between measures of overall morbidity for a population and measures associated with specific diseases or health conditions. Further, morbidity can be objectively measured (e.g., through clinical tests) or subjectively measured (e.g., through self-reports by individuals). While the morbidity level for the total population under study is important, it may be necessary to determine the morbidity level for subsets within the population (e.g., subgroups based on geography or demographic attribute) in order to truly understand a population's morbidity patterns.

Health

"Health" is perhaps one of the most difficult of healthcare terms related to morbidity to define. Not only is it a difficult concept to define in absolute terms, its meaning has changed over time. A variety of definitions have been proffered representing different perspectives, and none can be considered clearly right or wrong. As will be seen, the acceptable definition depends on one's perspective.

The very notion of health is a social ideal and its conceptualization varies widely from culture to culture and from one historical period to another. For example, in the nineteenth century the ideal upper-class woman in Europe was pale, frail, and delicate. A woman in robust health was considered to be lacking in refinement (Ehrenreich and English 1978). In other periods, cultures, or subcultures, however, the ideal of health might be identified with traits such as strength, fertility, righteousness, fatness, thinness, or youthfulness. Thus, a society's view of health embodies a particular that culture's notions of well-being and desired human qualities.

The Medical Model

There are a number of models for conceptualizing the concepts of health and illness (Wolinsky 1988). The historically dominant model in US society is the medical model. The *medical model* had its genesis in the establishment of germ theory as the basis for modern scientific medicine. This perspective emphasizes the existence of clearly identifiable clinical symptoms, reflecting the conviction that illness represents the existence of biological pathology. Thus illness is a state involving the presence of distinct symptoms; health is the negative residual condition reflecting an absence of symptoms.

Health and illness are conceptualized within this context in terms of biological "normality" and "abnormality." Health is considered the normal state, one free of any biological pathology. This view of health and illness continues to be widely accepted, since it is the view supported by mainstream medical practitioners. The manner in which most health problems are conceptualized and managed reflects this orientation, with both medical education and the organization of the healthcare system reinforcing this perspective. Health insurance constitutes an excellent example in that no treatment is covered without a physician's (i.e., a medical-model orientation) diagnosis.

As Freund and McGuire (1999) note, the medical model assumes a clear dichotomy between the mind and the body, with physical diseases presumed to be located within the body. The philosophical foundations for this mind/body dichotomy are often traced back to Descartes' division of the person into mind and body. The practical foundations, however, probably lie in medicine's shift to an emphasis on clinical observation toward the end of the eighteenth century and on pathological anatomy beginning in the nineteenth century. This notion implies that the body can be understood and treated in isolation from other aspects of the person inhabiting it (Hahn and Kleinman 1983). This medical perspective sees the body as docile—something physicians could observe, manipulate, transform, and improve. Diseases are conceptualized in terms of alterations in tissues that are visible upon opening the body, such as during autopsy.

The medical model further assumes that illness can be reduced to disordered bodily (biochemical or neurophysiological) functions. This physical reductionism excludes the social, psychological, and behavioral dimensions of illness (Engle 1977). The result of this reductionism, together with medicine's mind–body dualism, is that disease is localized within the individual body. Such conceptions prevent the medical model from considering any external factors that might impinge upon health.

A related assumption of the medical model is the belief that each disease is caused by a specific, presumably identifiable agent. This assumption arose from the nineteenth century work of Pasteur and Koch, who demonstrated that the introduction of specific virulent microorganisms (germs) into the body produced specific agents with a causal link to specific diseases. This doctrine of specific etiology was later extended beyond infectious diseases to a wide range of other conditions.

A variation of the medical model compares the body to a machine. From this perspective, disease represents the malfunctioning of some component of the "machine" (e.g., an organ). Modern medicine has not only retained the metaphor of the machine but also extended it by developing specializations along the lines of machine parts, emphasizing individual systems or organs to the exclusion of the totality of the body. The machine metaphor further encouraged an instrumentalist approach to the body; the physician could "repair" one part of the body in isolation from the rest (Berliner 1975). Health is, thus, the reflection of an efficiently functioning machine.

The medical model has been widely accepted because of its scientific basis and its usefulness in addressing certain types of disorders. It has been criticized, however, for its focus on acute rather than chronic conditions, its inability to account for nonphysical and/or asymptomatic conditions, and its reliance on professional "consensus" on what is considered normal and abnormal (Wolinsky 1988).

The Functional Model

A second approach to defining health and illness is referred to as the *functional model*. This model contends that health and illness reflect the level of *social* normality rather than physical normality characterizing an individual (Parsons 1972). This approach de-emphasizes the biologically based medical model in favor of a model based on social role performance. The healthy person is one who is able to function in keeping with society's expectations and is considered "normal" from a societal perspective. The absence of dysfunctional attributes indicates healthiness. The functional model is rooted in lay conceptualizations of health and illness rather than professional ones. From this perspective, the "diagnosis" is made by the social group based on societally based criteria rather than clinical ones. "Treatment" is geared toward restoring the affected individual to social normality rather than biological normality. The individual is seen as "cured" when he or she can resume social functioning, not when the clinical signs have disappeared.

Examples of the tension between the medical model and the functional model would include the alcoholic who, for years, is able to perform his job and maintain adequate family relationships. This person would be considered sick under the medical model but not under the functional model. Conversely, an individual complaining of chronic back pain would be considered sick under the functional model (assuming that the symptoms interfered with his or her social role performance), even if physicians could not identify any underlying pathological disorder. Another example would involve individuals with disabilities; an amputee, for example, who may be considered sick from the medical-model perspective but actually be capable of performing all required social roles.

The Psychological Model

Although the medical and functional models are considered the dominant paradigms, the *psychological model* should also be introduced (Antonovsky 1979). Alternately referred to as the "stress model," this is by far the most subjective of the three approaches. This model relies solely on self-evaluation by the individual for the determination of health and illness. If the individual feels well, he or she is well; if the same individual feels sick, he or she is sick. Similarly, only the affected party can determine when he or she is cured.

This approach focuses on the importance of stress in the production of sickness and argues that much of physical illness is a reaction to stress on the part of the individual. This perspective has gained some respect, now that the mind/body connection has been rediscovered and increasing emphasis is being placed on psychosomatic conditions. We now know, for example, that the effects of a positive attitude can be evidenced in every cell of the body as can the effects of a negative attitude. Further, we realize there are communities wherein all residents are exposed to constant stress with subsequent implications for health status.

The Legal Model

One final model that should be noted primarily applies to communicable diseases and mental illness. The *legal model* is applied in situations where the legal "health" or competence of the individual is in question. The ebola "scare" of 2014 reminds us of the importance of communicable disease control, and it is in this context that a legal definition of morbidity may come into play. Public health authorities have broad discretion when it comes to the containment of contagious diseases and the authority to declare a public health emergency if restrictions on travel and other social interaction are called for. Public health officials may even have priority over police in the management of individuals affected by some conditions, even something as common as sexually transmitted infections.

A legal definition also comes into play in cases where competence must be determined for involuntary hospital admission, guardianship, or custody decisions, and in cases where the individual's ability to manage his or her affairs is in question. Although a physician is generally required to certify the individual's competence, it is ultimately the courts that decide based on criteria established by the legal system. Thus, in the case of involuntary commitment, a psychiatrist must determine the extent to which the individual is a threat to himself or herself—or to others—and the extent to which he or she is competent to properly take care of himself or herself.

Although a psychiatrist performs the examination, the courts determine competence or incompetence in the final analysis.

The Biopsychosocial Model

One other definition of health that might be noted is the one formulated in the 1960s by the World Health Organization (WHO), the health arm of the United Nations. Health is defined by the WHO as a state of complete physical, psychological, social, and spiritual well-being and not merely the absence of disease and infirmity (World Health Organization 1999). While this rather idealistic definition was initially rejected as unworkable in the healthcare environment of the day, it has come to be accepted as the standard for defining health in contemporary society. Many Americans today expect to be healthy along all of the dimensions referenced in the WHO definition. It is ironic that American society has come to expect the scope of healthcare to extend far beyond the treatment of physical problems and into the management of psychological, social, and spiritual problems.

The modern view that many factors interact to produce health or ill-health may be attributed to the seminal work of George L. Engel, who put forward the *biopsychosocial model* of disease (Engle 1977). The biopsychosocial model takes a broad view of the factors that contribute to health and illness and argues that looking at biological factors alone—which was the prevailing view of disease at the time Engel was writing—is not sufficient to explain health and illness. According to Engel's model, biological, psychological, and social factors contribute to the causes, manifestation, course, and outcome of health and disease, including mental disorders. Few people with a condition such as heart disease or diabetes, for instance, would dispute the role of stress in aggravating their condition. Subsequent research supports the validity of this model.

Engel's model ultimately seeks to resolve the definitional dilemma by eliminating the either/or contention. It is not a matter of ill-health being caused by biological factors *or* social factors *or* psychological factors but rather a combination of the above. Everyone, it could be argued is exposed to disease organisms in the environment; this, however, is a necessary but not sufficient factor in the onset of disease. Other factors—social and/or emotional—may be required to trigger the disease episode. It is almost always the case with chronic conditions, in fact, that the condition results *only* through a combination of these three factors. Many people carry the indicator for rheumatoid arthritis in their blood, for example, but only a small proportion is affected. Those affected have typically had some social or psychological factors come into play that serve to activate the disease.

Ultimately, there is no *one* definition of "health." In fact, the definitions posed by health professionals may be quite different from lay definitions. (See Exhibit 2.1 for a discussion of the subjective nature of health and illness.) Each of the examples above may be appropriate for certain purposes under certain circumstances. Each has its advantages and disadvantages. As will be seen, the medical model has lost much of its salience as the epidemiological transition has shifted the burden of disease from acute conditions to chronic conditions.

Exhibit 2.1: The Subjective Nature of Morbidity

While we typically think the presence of illness is determined based on clinical measures, this objective depiction of ill-health is not the only manner in which illness is conceptualized. It is, in fact, a "modern" notion of the nature of illness. Societies (and even individuals) are likely to develop notions of health and illness that are particular to the situation and the social context. For that reason, it would not be unusual to find a disparity between the clinically identified conditions within a population and the conditions members of that population recognize. While biologically based health conditions are concrete and finite, socially defined conditions are more abstract and elastic. To understand the true level of morbidity within a population, both the objective and subjective dimensions need to be considered.

All things being equal, the absolute level of need should not vary much from population to population. Researchers working independently should draw the same conclusions with regard to the level and types of health conditions characterizing a specific population. This notion of an absolute level of morbidity relates more closely to the concept of biologically based "illness" than societally defined "sickness."

While epidemiologists are likely to find similar levels of morbidity from society to society, it is likely that the subjective levels will be quite different. Anthropologists tell us of societies where certain clearly identifiable diseases exist but society members insist that these are not manifestations of disease but while normal occurrenceswithin this population. Malnutrition that might be identified by a scientist within a population may be considered normal by that population. In our own, society, we have individuals who deny the existence of disease even though it may be clinically identifiable. While the detrimental effects of obesity have long been known, there are still segments of the US population that consider extreme overweight as a positive and even desirable state. Certainly, many Americans who could be diagnosed with a mental disorder would deny—perhaps based on the norms of their social group—that any such condition exists.

There are plenty of examples of societies' subjective view of illness that could be cited. Classic examples include the military induction center, where most prospective inductees are deemed disease free when there is high demand for servicemen but a "normal" amount of morbidity is discovered when there is no pressure on recruitment. Similarly, during the time of the Soviet Union, if a factory was not meeting its quota, the on-site physician might discover few cases of illness that would merit time off from work. On the other hand, if quotas were being met, a "normal" amount of morbidity was revealed.

The gap between "officially" defined morbidity and the level of morbidity perceived by any population will no doubt continue to be a fact of life. This situation must be kept in mind as definitions of health and ill-health are considered and the level of morbidity within the population discussed.

Ill-Health

While Americans appear to be obsessed with their health, it is the sickness aspect of the health/illness continuum that is the focus of our discussion and, indeed, the focus of the US healthcare system. The system's emphasis continues to be on sickness and not on health, despite all the press coverage the wellness movement has received over the past two decades. It is "sick" people, after all, that the healthcare delivery system was established to serve, leading some to refer to it as a system of "sick care" rather than "healthcare."

The condition of "ill-health" could be considered the converse of the state of health described above, although, as will be seen, this greatly oversimplifies the situation. Like health, its opposite can be defined in different ways depending on one's perspective. According to the medical model, illness involves the presence of clinically identifiable biological pathology. The focus of medical education and practice is on the presence of pathology—that is, biological abnormality—with little attention given to what constitutes a state of health and virtually no concern for the nonbiological factors involved in ill-health.

An important consideration in defining what constitutes ill-health involves the party that is responsible for this judgment. Under the medical model, a physician (and *only* a physician) can determine whether a person is sick or well. No treatment can be provided until a physician makes at least a provisional diagnosis, and the patient remains just that—a patient—until a physician pronounces him cured.

According to the functional model, ill-health involves a state of social abnormality. Individuals who do not or cannot comply with social norms related to role performance would be considered "ill" under this model. While the intent under the medical model is to return the affected individual to biological normality, actions taken within the context of the functional model attempt to restore social normality by allowing the affected individual to reassume appropriate social roles (regardless of his or her biological condition).

The process of identifying illness in a person unfolds differently in the functional model from the medical model. In the case of the former, there is no one "gatekeeper" to evaluate the state of the person's health. Representatives of that person's social group—reflecting the norms of the larger society—serve as "diagnosticians" and determine that the individual is not adequately functioning and is, thus, in ill health. Similarly, the social group concurs that the patient is cured when he or she is once again adequately carrying out prescribed social roles.

According to the psychological or stress model, the individual is considered in ill-health if the individual so defines himself. An individual who feels "disordered," out of sync with his social environment, or otherwise emotionally in disequilibrium would be considered in ill health under this model. This condition may manifest itself in physical or social abnormalities although the root cause is some internally based condition. In this case, only the affected individual can determine whether he or she is no longer "ill."

A situation in which the legal definition might be applied to physical illnesses would be in the case of certain "reportable" diseases and conditions requiring quarantine.

A test for a sexually transmitted infection that comes back positive makes the affected person legally ill and allows public health authorities to take action to bring about treatment and/or limit the spread of the disease.

In the case of involuntary committment to a mental institution, a psychiatrist must determine the extent to which the individual is a threat to himself–or to others–and/or the extent to which he is competent to properly take care of himself. The "judge" is generally not capable of making a judgment of "competence" but only "incompetence," with competence reflecting a lack of evidence for incompetence.

These questions highlight the fact that ill-health, like health, is essentially a social construct and may be viewed in different ways in different societies or even by different groups (including demographic subgroups) within the same society. Cultures and subcultures may vary in their perception of what constitutes ill-health, what physical states are symptomatic of morbidity, and what the significance of a particular morbid condition is.

Illness vs. Sickness

There are a number of terms used to describe ill-health, and the same term may be used in different ways under different circumstances. "Illness" and "sickness," for example, are terms used by demographers and the general public to describe ill-health. Although often used interchangeably, social scientists make a distinction between the two related concepts.

Illness refers to the individual, private, and, usually, biological aspect of ill-health. This perspective emphasizes the existence of clearly identifiable somatic symptoms, reflecting underlying biological pathology. Illness equates to the set of symptoms known primarily to the affected individual and in this sense is private as opposed to public. It is argued that illness (but not sickness) is a state shared by human beings with all other animals; that is, it is a state of biological dysfunction affecting the individual organism. The term may also be used to describe the condition that causes the ill-health (e.g., yellow fever is an illness that creates ill-health in the individual).

Cross-cultural studies of morbidity suggest that the level of illness is similar from society to society (Jurges 2007). All human populations share certain biological traits and, thus, the same susceptibility to certain diseases. Thus, it could be argued that differences in the morbidity patterns of a particular population are mostly a function of time and place. All things being equal, one could expect the same level of morbidity from one population to another in terms of the number of extant conditions, the differences being a function of the types of conditions common to the respective populations.

Sickness refers to the public or social component of ill-health. Illness is transformed into sickness when the condition becomes publicly known through announcement by the affected party, observation by significant others, or professional diagnosis. Thus, while illness is primarily a biological state, sickness is a social state. Sickness is social not only because it is recognized beyond the bounds of the individual but also because it has implications for social role performance and interpersonal interaction.

The transition from a state of illness to a state of sickness has implications for both the individual and the social group. Once the individual's condition becomes public the affected individual begins to see himself in a different light. Social relationships may be modified and social interactions affected. The person's self-concept is likely to undergo modification as he accepts the group's acknowledgement of his abnormality. At the same time, the social group comes to view the affected party in a different light. The individual is no longer able to perform valued social roles, is exempt from certain responsibilities, and may be consuming valuable societal resources. The affected individual cannot meet the expectations of society until he is restored to a state of normal functioning.

Unlike illness, the level of sickness varies widely from society to society and within the same society over time. Since the amount of sickness reflects the perceptions of society, a list of common sicknesses would vary from society to society. This means that the level of sickness is much more "elastic" than the level of illness, with the amount of sickness rising or falling based on changing social circumstances.

Physical Illness and Mental Illness

A distinction is made within the scientific community and by the general public between physical illness and mental illness. Because of this distinction, the US healthcare system addresses physical illness and mental illness quite differently, and the emergence of allopathic medicine in the twentieth century served to formalize the distinction between physical disorders and mental disorders.

Traditional societies typically viewed all illnesses under the same umbrella. Whatever the form of the malady, it was thought to be a function of disequilibrium on the part of the individual, the intervention of some supernatural force, or some other phenomenon of unknown origin. Differential diagnosis (i.e., the precise classification of disease) was not emphasized, and the etiology (i.e., the cause or source) of the problem was the main consideration in evaluating a symptomatic individual.

Modern Western thinking led to a clear distinction between the physical and the mental domains. This perspective was reinforced by the entrenchment of germ theory in the medical model paradigm. The biomedical model's emphasis on biological causes led to the separation of conditions that demonstrated clear biological pathology (physical illnesses) from those that did not (mental illnesses). This distinction is reflected in what is essentially a separate sector within the healthcare system for the treatment of mental disorders, complete with distinct facilities and practitioners. A clear distinction is maintained today between mental hospitals and general hospitals and, in medical practice, between psychiatrists and other physicians.

Physical illness and mental illness do differ from each other in a number of ways. Physical illness is generally characterized by clear-cut, clinically identifiable symptoms, while mental illness is not. The symptoms of physical illness reflect biological pathology while those of mental illness are more likely to reflect disorders of mood, behavior, and thought. Thus, the diagnosis of most mental disorders is more subjective than that of physical disorders because of the lack of clinical diagnostic tests. Although a small portion of mental disorders can be attributed to some underlying biological pathology (e.g., nervous system damage), most mental conditions are thought to reflect either internal psychological pathology or the influence of external stressors (Scull 2015). Neither of these lends itself to traditional medical diagnostic techniques.

The definitions of mental health and illness reflect the same models or perspectives associated with physical health and illness. The medical model remains important, primarily due to the pivotal role of the psychiatrist in diagnosis and treatment. However, the functional model is particularly relevant in that mental pathology is more likely to be identified based on some functional impairment rather than a biological impairment. Indeed, most cases of mental disorder go undetected until social relationships are so disrupted that a response is required. Ironically, the psychological model probably has the least salience in that it assumes the individual making an assessment of healthiness is in his or her "right mind." It should also be remembered that mental health or illness is sometimes defined from a legal perspective. The courts may be placed in the position of determining the mental capacity of the effected individual.

Mental illness also differs from physical illness in that most mental disorders are considered to be both chronic and incurable. The basic goal of medicine is the treatment and cure of disease, yet most mental disorders are considered to be permanent and not amenable to cure. They can only be managed. This makes the medical model of limited usefulness as a framework for viewing mental illness.

Mental illness is also perceived much differently by the general public than is physical illness. Mental illness carries more of a stigma than do most physical illnesses; one can recover from the latter it is believed, but not necessarily from the former. At the same time, the unpredictability of the behavior of the mentally ill tends to make the "normal" person uncomfortable in the face of psychiatric symptoms. Exhibit 2.2 discusses issues surrounding the definition of psychiatric morbidity.

Disability

Another term used to define morbidity is *disability*. In many ways, disability is even more difficult to operationalize than other morbidity concepts. "Disability" refers to any short- or long-term reduction of a person's activity as a result of an acute or chronic condition. While it would appear simple to enumerate the blind, deaf, or otherwise handicapped, the situation is actually quite complex. Does lower back pain that interferes with work constitute a disability? When does an arthritic condition become disabling? How is mental retardation classified, and at what point? Even those disabilities that appear obvious defy easy categorization due to the subjective dimension of disability. There are many hearing impaired individuals and amputees, for example, that would take exception to being classified as disabled.

The dominance of the medical model has led to an acute care approach to disability. However, such a framework offers an inadequate view of disability for a number of reasons. Acute care perspectives are primarily restricted to somatic conditions, yet contemporary concepts of disability include conditions that may not exhibit physical signs or symptoms. Disability may limit an individual's capacity to live independently or care for him- or herself; it may interfere with maintaining or initiating relationships, pursuing career goals, or enjoying leisure activities. The effects of nonphysical injuries such as post-traumatic stress disorder (PTSD) have had to be increasingly considered.

Increasing attention has also been paid to developmental disabilities. Developmental disabilities are a diverse group of severe chronic conditions that are due to mental and/or physical impairments. People with developmental disabilities have problems with major life activities such as language, mobility, learning, self-help, and independent living. Developmental disabilities begin anytime during development up to 22 years of age and usually last throughout a person's lifetime.

As a result of the challenges involved in defining disability in terms of specific handicaps, it has become common to conceptualize disability based on the consequences of a condition. In the National Health Interview Survey conducted by the National Center for Health Statistics, for example, "limitation of activity" refers to a long-term reduction due to a chronic condition in a person's capacity to perform the usual kind or amount of activities associated with his or her age group. Limitation of activity is assessed by asking respondents a series of questions about their ability to perform activities usual for people their age. These include inquiries on limitations in activities related to daily living, instrumental tasks, play, school or work, walking or remembering. With this approach, disability is assessed based on some type of limitation scale or in terms of days of restricted activity.

Exhibit 2.2: The Special Case of Psychiatric Morbidity

Mental illness is not diagnosed in the same manner as other chronic diseases. Heart disease is identified with the help of blood tests and electrocardiograms. Diabetes is diagnosed by measuring blood glucose levels. But diagnosing mental illness is a more subjective endeavor. No blood test exists for depression; no X-ray can identify a child at risk of developing bipolar disorder. Today, however, new tools in genetics and neuroimaging are assisting in deciphering details of the underlying biology of mental disorders, raising questions about the nature of mental disorders. For example, are mental illnesses simply physical diseases that happen to strike the brain...or do these disorders belong in a class all their own?

One school of thought insists that it all comes down to biology. This approach emphasizes the role of physical abnormalities in creating mental disorders, an approach championed by many at the National Institute of Mental Health. This orientation contends that mental illnesses are no different from heart disease, diabetes, or any other chronic illness. All chronic diseases have behavioral components as well as biological components, with the organ of interest here the brain instead of the heart or pancreas. This perspective argues that we are at the point with regard to mental illness that we were with cardiology a century ago when, as in the case of mental disorders, there were no clinical tests to determine the nature and extent of heart conditions. This does not eliminate the

(continued)

Exhibit 2.2 (continued)

behavioral component but suggests the need for a toolkit that indicates what is going on from the behavioral level to the molecular level.

In recent years scientists have made numerous discoveries about the function—and dysfunction—of the human brain. Genes linked to schizophrenia have been identified and brain abnormalities that increase a person's risk of developing post-traumatic stress disorder after a distressing event have been discovered. Researchers have also begun to flesh out a physiological explanation for depression. Understanding the underlying biology helps therapists and psychopharmacologists decide which type of treatment patients would benefit from.

Despite these advances most experts concede that some mental illnesses will never be described in purely biological terms, especially since it is impossible to control all variables that might influence mental health status. One of the biggest problems is that mental illness diagnoses are often catchall categories that include many different underlying malfunctions. Mental illnesses have always been described by their outward symptoms, both out of necessity and convenience. But just as cancer patients are a diverse group marked by many different disease pathways, a depression diagnosis is likely to encompass people with many unique underlying problems. That presents challenges for defining the disease in biological terms.

When it comes to mental illness, a one-size-fits-all approach does not apply. Some diseases may be more purely physiological in nature. For example, schizophrenia, bipolar disorder, and autism fit the biological model in a very clear-cut sense. In these diseases structural and functional abnormalities are evident in imaging scans or during postmortem dissection. Yet for other conditions, such as depression or anxiety, the biological foundation is more nebulous. Mental illnesses are likely to have multiple causes, including genetic, biological, and environmental factors, and our understanding of the interplay among those factors is nowhere near as well developed as it is for many chronic diseases. The danger in placing too much attention on the biological is that important environmental, behavioral, and social factors that contribute to mental illness may be overlooked.

This has led some to argue that too much emphasis is being placed on the biology of mental illness at this point in our understanding of the brain. Decades of effort to understand the biology of mental disorders have uncovered clues, but those clues haven't translated into improvements in diagnosis or treatment. Some conditions may even stem from a chance combination of normal personality traits. While the brain circuitry is equivalent to the hardware, we also have the human equivalent of software. Just as software bugs are often the cause of our computer problems, our mental motherboards can be done in by our psychological processing.

Source: Weir, Kristen (2012). The roots of mental illness. *Monitor on Psychology* 43(June):6.

Mortality as a Proxy for Morbidity

In the past, it has been common to use mortality data as a proxy for morbidity data. Historically, there was a fairly close correlation between common maladies and common causes of death. The immediate cause of death was typically the primary cause of death, with few complicating factors involved. Further, mortality data have long been relatively complete and easily attainable. The connection between mortality and morbidity can still be made today to a certain extent, in that the leading causes of death (heart disease and cancer) reflect common maladies within the population.

Over time, however, the mortality rate has become a less meaningful proxy for morbidity. In the US the mortality rate has dropped to the point that death is a relatively rare event. Further, the correspondence between mortality and morbidity has become diminished. Because of the preponderance of chronic disease within the US population, death certificates are less and less likely to capture the underlying disease. Chronic diseases typically do not kill people, but some complication (of diabetes, AIDS, or cancer, for example) is typically the proximate cause of death. This is not to say that mortality analysis cannot provide insights into morbidity patterns, but that the situation is much more complicated than in the past, and contemporary analyses of mortality data require a better understanding of disease processes (and the vagaries of death certificates). In subsequent sections, reference will be made to mortality as a proxy for morbidity with, however, the caveats expressed here. Exhibit 2.3 discusses the fluid nature of conditions considered morbid.

Exhibit 2.3: The Fluid Definition of Morbid Conditions

The study of morbidity is complicated by the fact that what is classified as illness can change over time. These changes may result from a number of factors—diseases being eradicated (e.g., small pox), conditions being renamed or reclassified (e.g., homosexuality), newly discovered conditions (e.g., Legionnaire's disease), or a newly recognized condition (e.g., adolescent adjustment disorder). Some of this results from the emergence of truly new conditions recognized by health professionals. These could be newly emergent conditions such as human immunodeficiency virus (HIV) or antibiotic-resistant influenza. Or they could be newly introduced conditions that previously existed outside the US.

It is often the case that a nonclinical condition becomes redefined as a clinical condition. A symptom or set of symptoms that is common within a population may come to be defined as a disease. The management of pregnancy is a case in point. Historically pregnancy (and childbirth) was considered a natural process that should involve clinical attention only if a complication occurs. In the twentieth century pregnancy came to be seen as a

(continued)

Exhibit 2.3 (continued)

medical condition that required the attention of the healthcare system before, during, and after childbirth.

A number of "new" conditions have been similarly identified over time and added to the list of diseases affecting the US population. Among the conditions involving previously existing syndromes that have been newly added to the accepted list of clinical conditions are:

- Attention deficit hyperactivity disorder
- Adjustment disorder
- Irritable bowel syndrome
- Autism
- Obesity
- Menopause
- Premenstrual syndrome
- Chronic fatigue syndrome
- Post-traumatic stress disorder

It should be noted that none of these are actually new conditions but each involved symptoms that had not previously thought to reflect morbid states. They may have been accepted as normal aspects of living (e.g., hyperactivity in kids now identified as "ADHD") or considered an understandable consequence of an experience (e.g., soldiers suffering from shellshock now defined as "post-traumatic stress disorder").

There are other albeit less common examples of conditions being identified as morbid states in the past but now considered "normal" or at least not a morbid condition. For example, in the past alcohol abuse was classified as a disease and is still considered a psychiatric condition in the diagnostic manual used by mental health professionals. However, the contention that there was an underlying biological basis for alcoholism has been mostly rejected in favor of a more behaviorist explanation to alcohol abuse. Homosexuality is another condition whose status has evolved over time. At one time, homosexuality was officially identified as a medical condition and treated as such by the medical community. If not resulting from a biological defect, it was considered to be a serious psychiatric condition. The thinking has evolved to reflect a more contemporary perception of homosexuality and it has been removed from the list of "diseases."

It is beyond the scope of this work to judge the merits of redefining commonly occurring states as morbid conditions or the motives for some of these reclassifications. The main point is that there are few absolutes when it comes to defining syndromes or states as diseases. Various syndromes may be defined as diseases in various places at various points in time. At the same time, conditions long accepted as pathological (e.g., "hysteria" in women) may be discarded as unworthy of the disease classification.

Other Useful Concepts

Acute Conditions

Health conditions are typically classified as either acute or chronic. An acute condition is a health condition characterized by rapid onset, usually short duration, and a
clear-cut disposition (e.g., recovery, death). A more technical definition is utilized
by the National Center for Health Statistics and reads: An acute condition is a type
of illness or injury that ordinarily lasts less than 3 months, was first noticed less than
3 months before the date of data collection, and was serious enough to have had an
impact on behavior. Pregnancy is considered to be an acute condition despite lasting
longer than 3 months. Common acute conditions include respiratory problems,
communicable diseases, parasitic diseases, gastrointestinal problems, and
accidents.

Acute conditions are the dominant type of health problem in traditional societies
(e.g., hunting-and-gathering, agricultural societies) and developing countries, and
virtually everyone within these populations is at the same risk of morbidity. Younger
populations are also more likely to be characterized by acute conditions with the
prevalence of such conditions declining with age. Limited public health facilities,
impoverishment, and a young age structure all contribute to a predominance of
acute conditions. Further, the short average life expectancy characterizing some
populations mitigates against the appearance of many chronic conditions—that is,
people do not live long enough to develop conditions that reflect years of cumulative
wear or old age.

Chronic Conditions

A chronic condition is a health condition characterized by slow onset, lengthy progression, and a usually indefinite disposition, typical of modern, industrial societies.
The National Center for Health Statistics considers a health condition to be chronic
if it lasts more than 3 months. Common chronic conditions include arthritis, cardiovascular disease, cancer, diabetes, epilepsy and seizures, and obesity. Conditions
that are not cured once acquired (such as heart disease, diabetes, and birth defects)
are considered chronic. An exception is made for children less than 1 year of age
who have had a condition "since birth," as these conditions are always considered
chronic.

Chronic conditions are common in more industrialized societies and in those
with an older age structure. The acute conditions common to younger populations
are supplanted by chronic conditions that reflect lifestyles, health behaviors and the
accumulative effect of a life of stress and wear and tear. In populations where
chronic conditions predominate a significant portion of the population is likely to be
affected since, unlike acute conditions, chronic conditions do not go away. The

CDC reports that today more than half of the US population is affected by at least one chronic disease (National Center for Health Statistics 2013). Exhibit 2.4 presents a comparison of the attributes of acute and chronic conditions. Exhibit 2.5 provides a case study in the identification of a "new" disease.

Exhibit 2.4: Characteristics of Acute and Chronic Conditions

	Acute condition	Chronic condition
Etiology	Simple/singular	Complex/multiple
Rate of onset	Rapid	Slow/insidious
Distinctiveness of onset	Clear-cut	Difficult to diagnose
Duration of illness	Short-lived	Perpetual
Treatment	Counter pathogens	Manage symptoms
Course of disease	Recovery or death	Slow progression
Goal of care	Cure	Management
Duration of care	Short-term	Lifelong
Contribution to mortality	Direct	Indirect

Source: Thomas, Richard K. (2005). Society and Health: Sociology for Health Professionals. New York: Springer

Comorbidity

Comorbidity refers to the concurrent existence of two or more disease processes. The term is used both to refer to conditions that exist simultaneously but independently within a single patient and to a condition that is caused by the primary condition. It is also used to refer to the state produced by the presence of of comorbidity. There is no "official" definition of comorbidity and it is defined differently by different parties.

In the mental health arena, comorbidity refers to the presence of more than one diagnosis occurring in an individual at the same time. In psychiatry, comorbidity does not necessarily imply the presence of multiple diseases, but instead can reflect our current inability to supply a single diagnosis that accounts for all symptoms. Psychiatric comorbidity is often found in those with addictions, major depressive disorders, and personality disorders.

Comorbidity is a common characteristic of patients, with some observers considering it the norm rather than the exception. Autopsies often reveal the existence of comorbidities that were undiagnosed in the living person. With the ascendancy of chronic diseases within the US population, the number of patients with comorbidities has increased. This is due to both the independent emergence of conditions among older patients (e.g., heart disease, arthritis, and glaucoma) and the spillover effect of another chronic condition (e.g., blindness or amputation caused by diabetes).

Exhibit 2.5: The Discovery of a New Disease: The Case of Menopause

A variety of factors may contribute to the discovery of a "new" disease. This may involve the identification of a here-to-fore unknown condition (e.g., Legionnaire's disease or AIDS) and the subsequent classification and naming of it. It may involve the discovery of a syndrome involving a set of symptoms not previously connected (e.g., Alzheimer's disease). Or it may involve the redefinition of an existing condition as a health problem (e.g., alcoholism).

The last means of disease recognition is relevant to menopause which was added to the list of diseases in the *International Classification of Diseases* in the 1980s. Although menopause is considered to be a normal biological process, it has become increasingly "medicalized" over the past 50 years. During this period, the condition was transformed from symptoms that were essentially "all in the head" of affected women to a clinical condition involving estrogen deficiency or ovarian dysfunction.

Despite the universality of menopause among women regardless of the society, there are remarkable differences in the biophysical, social, and emotional dimensions of the condition from culture to culture. However, the social connotations and expectations associated with menopause are mostly ignored by modern Western medicine. The condition is reduced to a set of biochemical processes presumed to characterize all female bodies, regardless of social or cultural context. The notion of menopause as a pathological condition originated with a specific body of research but, once the condition was isolated, the "disease" took on a life of its own unaffected by subsequent research.

Early research, for example, was based on women who had experienced surgically induced menopause or who suffered from extreme conditions that involved unusual physical side effects. The findings drawn from an abnormal population were extrapolated to the general population, and the notion of menopause as a disease became firmly entrenched. More recent research utilizing "normal" subjects has found no evidence of pathology or medical problems. Not only do most women not experience abnormal symptoms but, among the few who do, there are typically other health problems accompanying the onset of menopause. Thus, it could be argued that other health conditions contribute to problem menopause and not the other way around.

To a great extent, the identification of menopause as a pathological condition was a result of a "campaign" by a handful of endocrinologists who were proponents of menopause as a hormonal disorder during the 1930s and 1940s. Other physicians were willing to accept this notion because if fit well with their medical model concept of disease. As is often the case, the identification of a syndrome as a disease was facilitated by the availability of a "cure" (in this case inexpensive synthetic estrogen). Not only could a pathological state be identified, but a medical treatment had become available for its management. Thus, despite the fact that 15 % or less of American women experienced

(continued)

Exhibit 2.5 (continued)

problem menopause, in 1975 it was found that 51 % of women had taken estrogen replacement drugs at some point.

Despite the risks now known to be associated with estrogen replacement therapy, the medical community continues to debate the existence of menopause as a disease. The fact that there are proponents on both sides of the issue reminds us that the formal identification of a disease is often a function of the perspectives of the health professionals involved. It could be argued, in fact, that there are very few diseases in an absolute sense, with the identification of disease being as much a social phenomenon as a clinical one.

References

Antonovsky, A. (1979). *Health, stress and coping*. San Francisco: Jossey-Bass.

Berliner, H. S. (1975). A larger perspective on the Flexner report. *International Journal of Health Services, 5*, 573–592.

Ehrenreich, B., & English, D. (1978). *For her own good: 150 of the experts' advice to women*. Garden City, NY: Doubleday.

Engle, G. L. (1977). The need for a new medical model: A challenge for biomedicine. *Science, 196*, 129–135.

Freund, P. E. S., & McGuire, M. B. (1999). *Health, illness and the social body* (3rd ed.). Englewood Cliffs, NJ: Prentice Hall.

Hahn, R. A., & Kleinman, A. (1983). Biomedical practice and anthropological theory: Frameworks and directions. *Annual Review of Anthropology, 12*, 305–333.

Jurges, H. (2007). True health vs. response styles: Exploring cross-country differences in self-reported health status. *Health Economics, 16*(2), 163–178.

National Center for Health Statistics. (2013). *Chronic diseases: The power to prevent, the call to control*. Retrieved April 1, 2013, from http://www.cdc.gov/chronicdisease/resources/publications/aag/chronic.htm.

Parsons, T. (1972). Definitions of health and illness in the light of American values and social structure. In E. G. Jaco (Ed.), *Patients, physicians, and illness* (pp. 107–127). New York: MacMillan.

Scull, A. (2015). *Madness in civilization: A cultural history of insanity from the Bible to Freud, from the madhouse to modern medicine*. Princeton, NJ: Princeton University Press.

Thomas, R. K. (2005). *Society and health: Sociology for health professionals*. New York: Springer.

Weir, K. (2012). The roots of mental illness. *Monitor on Psychology, 43*(June), 6.

Wolinsky, F. D. (1988). *The sociology of health: Principles, professions, and issues* (2nd ed.). Belmont, CA: Wadsworth.

World Health Organization (1999). Retrieved from www.who.int/aboutwho/en/definition.html.

Additional Resources

Gordis, L. (2008). *Epidemiology* (4th ed.). Philadelphia: Saunders.

Haubrich, W. S. (1984). *Medical meanings: A glossary of word origins*. New York: Harcourt Brace Jovanovich.

www.cdc.gov. Primary federal source of information on morbidity.

www.medicinenet.com. On-line medical dictionary.

Chapter 3
Categories of Morbidity Data

Introduction

The classification of objects in the world, whether natural or manmade, is a prerequisite for both the rational explanation of any phenomena and the development of science. Medical science, especially the contemporary Western version, is highly dependent on classification systems or disease nosology, and a number of classifications systems are utilized to categorize health conditions. From a practical standpoint, epidemiologists, medical practitioners, and healthcare administrators must be able to place health conditions into appropriate categories for a variety of reasons, and the relevant system depends on the intended purposes. For example, the system used to classify physical illness differs from that used to classify mental illness.

Most existing classification systems were established to facilitate the diagnostic process. Subsequently, these classification systems have come to be used for administrative, planning, and fiscal management purposes. Administrators need to organize the delivery of care around the categories of health problems that must be addressed. Planners must be able to anticipate the types of services that will be needed in the future. Financial managers must be able to specify the diagnoses affecting patients in order to determine the cost of care and the charges to be levied for the services provided.

In addressing the issue of "the categories" a distinction should be made between morbidity associated with an individual (clinical morbidity) and morbidity associated with a group (epidemiological morbidity). This distinction reflects the unresolved issue of whether researchers should consider morbidity at the individual level or at an aggregate level. This and subsequent discussions will focus on morbidity as an attribute of a population independent for the most part of the morbidity of individuals.

© Springer New York 2016
R.K. Thomas, *In Sickness and In Health*, Applied Demography Series 6,
DOI 10.1007/978-1-4939-3423-2_3

Despite the presumed objectivity of medical science, the development of a workable disease classification system has been challenging. The use of modern diagnostic techniques and sophisticated biomedical testing equipment has complicated the classification of disease as ever finer distinctions can be made between various syndromes. Part of the problem stems from controversy over exactly how "disease" should be defined. The reality is that disease syndromes are not necessarily clear-cut and mutually exclusive, diagnostic tests are far from precise, and conventional standards for defining diseases tend to shift in accordance with new research findings, new treatment modalities, and even nonclinical developments. These problems—and the concomitant criticisms—are exacerbated when attempts are made at classifying disabilities or mental disorders. The systems that have been developed, therefore, although widely used, are not without their critics. Although less than perfect, these existing classification systems provide the framework within which medical science operates.

The Classification of Physical Illnesses

Most disease classification systems focus on physical illness rather than mental illness (although there is some overlap between the two types of systems). The section below describes commonly employed disease classification systems for physical illnesses (including injuries and disabilities) with mental illness classification discussed in a later section.

International Classification of Diseases

The most widely recognized and utilized disease classification system is the *International Classification of Diseases*. The International Classification of Diseases (ICD) system, whose major disease categories are shown in Exhibit 3.1, is the official classificatory scheme developed by the World Health Organization within the United Nations. The version currently utilized in the US is ICD-9-CM, with CM standing for "clinical modification" (Centers for Disease Control and Prevention 2015). The US version reflects modifications necessary in keeping with current medical practice in American hospitals. (An updated version of the ICD system—version 10—has been developed and is slowly being introduced.)

The ICD system is designed for the classification of morbidity and mortality information and for the indexing of diseases and procedures that occur within a clinical setting. The present classification system includes two components: diagnoses and procedures. Two different sets of codes are assigned to the respective components; the codes are detailed enough that very fine distinctions can be made between various syndromes and procedures.

Originally, the ICD system was designed to facilitate worldwide communication concerning diseases, to provide a basis for statistical record-keeping and epidemiological studies, and to facilitate research into the quality of healthcare. However, additional functions have evolved in which the system is used to facilitate payment for health services, evaluate utilization patterns, and study the appropriateness of healthcare costs.

The disease classification component (found in volumes 1 and 2) utilizes 17 disease and injury categories, along with two "supplementary" classifications. Within each of these major categories, specific conditions are listed in detail. A three-digit number is assigned to the various major subdivisions within each of the 17 categories. These three-digit numbers are extended another digit to indicate the subcategory within the larger category (in order to add clinical detail or isolate terms for clinical accuracy). A fifth digit is sometimes added to further specify any factors associated with that particular diagnosis. For example, Hodgkin's disease, a form of malignant neoplasm or cancer, is coded as 201. A particular type of Hodgkin's disease, Hodgkin's sarcoma, is coded 201.2. If the Hodgkin's sarcoma affects the lymph nodes of the neck, it is coded 201.21.

The supplementary classifications are a concession to the fact that many non-medical factors are involved in the onset of disease, responses to disease, and utilization of services. These additional codes attempt to identify causes of disease or injury states that are external to the biophysical system. Exhibit 3.1 presents the major categories of diseases and injuries recognized within the ICD classification system. Exhibit 3.2 provides an example of the classification of a particular condition.

Exhibit 3.1: Major Categories of Diseases and Injuries

International Classification of Diseases Version 9	
1	Infectious and parasitic diseases
2	Neoplasms
3	Endocrine, nutritional, and metabolic diseases and immunity disorders
4	Diseases of the blood and blood-forming organs
5	Mental diseases
6	Diseases of the nervous system and sense organs
7	Diseases of the circulatory system
8	Diseases of the respiratory system
9	Diseases of the digestive system
10	Diseases of the genitourinary system
11	Complications of pregnancy, childbirth, and the puerperium
12	Diseases of the skin and subcutaneous tissue
13	Diseases of the musculoskeletal system and connective tissues
14	Congenital anomalies
15	Certain conditions originating in the perinatal period
16	Symptoms, signs, and ill-defined conditions
17	Injury and poisoning
V	Classification of factors influencing health status and contact with health service
E	Classification of external causes of injury and poisoning

Diagnostic Related Groups

Efforts aimed at slowing healthcare expenditures were initiated during the 1980s by the federal government in response to the financial demands placed on the Medicare program, the Medicaid program, and other federally supported healthcare initiatives. The most significant step in this regard was the introduction of "prospective payment" as the basis for reimbursement for health services rendered under the Medicare program. Reimbursement is determined by the Diagnostic Related Group (DRG) that is assigned to the hospital episode. Under this arrangement, hospitals, physicians, and certain other providers of health services are informed at the beginning of the financial accounting period of the amount that the federal government will pay for a particular category of patient as determined by their classification into one of 753 DRGs (Advance Healthcare 2015). This is in stark contrast to the "retrospective payment" approach originally built into the Medicare program, which was essentially a cost- plus arrangement with no incentives for cost containment. The prospective payment system (PPS) limits the amount of reimbursement for service to each category of patient based on rates predetermined by the Centers for Medicare and Medicaid Services (CMS), the federal agency that administers the Medicare program.

Exhibit 3.2: Example of Disease Classification Using ICD-9-CM

Condition	Code
Ischemic heart disease	410–414
Coronary atherosclerosis	414.0
Aneurysm of heart	414.1
Aneurysm of heart wall	414.10
Aneurysm of coronary vessels	414.11
Other aneurysm	414.12
Other specified forms of chronic ischemic heart disease	414.8
Chronic ischemic heart disease, not elsewhere specified	414.9

Introduced by the federal government during the 1980s, DRGs represented an attempt to standardize the classification of hospital patients whose care was being financed by the Medicare program. DRGs represent a mixture of diagnoses and procedures. The primary diagnosis is modified by such factors as coexisting conditions, presence of complications, patient's age, and usual length of hospital stay in order to create the 753 diagnostic categories currently in use. Exhibit 3.3 presents a sampling of DRGs along with their codes.

Exhibit 3.3: Example Diagnostic Related Groups

DRG code	DRG description
071	Nonspecific cerebrovascular disorders with complications
072	Nonspecific cerebrovascular disorders without complications
073	Cranial and peripheral nerve disorders with major complications
074	Cranial and peripheral nerve disorders without major complications
075	Viral meningitis with complications
076	Viral meningitis without complications
077	Hypertensive encephalopathy with major complications
078	Hypertensive encephalopathy with complications
079	Hypertensive encephalopathy without complications
080	Nontraumatic stupor and coma
082	Traumatic stupor and coma
088	Concussion with major complications
089	Concussion with complications
090	Concussion without complications
091	Other disorders of nervous system with major complications
092	Other disorders of nervous system with complications
093	Other disorders of nervous system without complications
095	Bacterial and tuberculous infections of the nervous system with complications
096	Bacterial and tuberculous infections of the nervous system without complications

DRGs can be grouped into 25 major diagnostic categories (MDCs) in order to simplify the system. These MDCs are based primarily on the different body systems. MDCs may be used when a broader view of disease categories is desirable. Exhibit 3.4 lists the MDCs currently in use.

Exhibit 3.4: Major Diagnostic Categories for Diagnostic Related Groups

MDC code	MDC description
1	Nervous system
2	Eye
3	Ear, nose, mouth, and throat
4	Respiratory system
5	Circulatory system
6	Digestive system
7	Hepatobiliary system and pancreas
8	Musculoskeletal system and connective tissue

(continued)

Exhibit 3.4 (continued)

MDC code	MDC description
9	Skin, subcutaneous tissue, and breast
10	Endocrine, nutritional, and metabolic system
11	Kidney and urinary tract
12	Male reproductive system
13	Female reproductive system
14	Pregnancy, childbirth, and puerperium
15	Newborn and other neonates
16	Blood and blood-forming organs and immunological disorders
17	Myeloproliferative disorders
18	Infectious and parasitic disorders
19	Mental disease and disorders
20	Alcohol/drug use of induced mental disorders
21	Injuries, poison, and toxic effect of drugs
22	Burns
23	Factors influencing health status
24	Multiple significant trauma
25	Human immunodeficiency virus infection

Reportable or Notifiable Disease Classification

"Reportable" conditions, or notifiable diseases, represent another system of disease classification. Within the US, each state has the authority to define conditions of public health importance, also known as State Reportable Conditions, with the list of such conditions varying from state to state. "Notifiable" conditions are those that are recognized as reportable across all states and territories (Centers for Disease Control and Prevention 2014). The Centers for Disease Control and Prevention (CDC) and the Council of State and Territorial Epidemiologists (CSTE) designate certain conditions as nationally notifiable (also called National Notifiable Conditions or NNCs).

A condition might be on the national list but not be reportable in a particular state. In addition, conditions may be on a state's list of State Reportable Conditions that are not on the national list. Each state carries the authority to determine which conditions reporting entities (laboratories, hospitals, healthcare providers, etc.) are required to report. This discussion focuses on notifiable diseases since this list is standard for all public health authorities.

The CDC requests that states notify them when an instance of a disease or condition occurs that meets the national case definition. Potential (suspect) cases of notifiable diseases are reported to local, regional, or state public health authorities. These reports might be based on a positive laboratory test, clinical symptoms, or epidemiologic criteria. A public health investigation is sometimes conducted to determine the need for appropriate public health interventions. When a suspect case is determined to meet the national case definition, de-identified data are sent to the CDC. This can include information reported to public health authorities by laboratories and healthcare providers, along with other information collected during public health investigations.

Notifiable diseases have been singled out primarily because of their communicable nature and for which regular, frequent, and timely information on individual cases is considered necessary for the prevention and control of the disease. Public health officials are particularly interested in conditions that have the potential to spread to epidemic proportions. It should be noted that virtually all notifiable diseases are acute conditions, at a time when chronic conditions represent the dominant health threat. For this reason, notifiable morbid conditions have become less useful over time as indicators of health status.

The list of nationally notifiable diseases is revised periodically and currently there are 52 infectious diseases so designated at the national level. A disease may be added to the list as a new pathogen emerges, or a disease may be deleted as its incidence declines. Public health officials at state health departments and the CDC continue to collaborate in determining which diseases should be nationally notifiable. The CSTE, with input from the CDC, makes recommendations annually for additions and deletions to the list of nationally notifiable diseases. Reporting is currently mandated (i.e., by state legislation or regulation) only at the state level and the reporting of data on notifiable diseases to the CDC is voluntary. All states generally report the internationally quarantinable diseases (e.g., cholera, plague, and yellow fever) in compliance with the World Health Organization's International Health Regulations.

Data on notifiable diseases are available from the CDC in all 50 states, the District of Columbia, and 122 selected cities. The data are available on a monthly basis in *Morbidity and Mortality Weekly Report*, a CDC publication, and at http://www2.cdc.gov:81/mmwr/mmwr.htm. Additional information on notifiable diseases can be found at http://www.cdc.gov. Exhibit 3.5 presents the current (2013) list of notifiable diseases.

Exhibit 3.5: Infectious Diseases Designated as Notifiable at the National Level: 2013

Anthrax
Arboviral diseases
Babesiois
Botulism
Brucellosis
Chancroid
Chlamydia trachomatis infection
Cholera
Coccidioidomycosis
Cryptosporidiosis
Cyclosporiasis
Dengue virus infection
Diphtheria
Ehrlichiosis/Anaplasmosis
Giardiasis

(continued)

Exhibit 3.5   (continued)

Gonorrhea
Haemophilus influenzae, invasive disease
Hansen disease (leprosy)
Hantavirus pulmonary syndrome
Hemolytic uremic syndrome, post-diarrheal
Hepatitis, viral
Human immunodeficiency virus (HIV) infection
Influenza-associated pediatric mortality
Legionellosis
Listeriosis
Lyme disease
Malaria
Measles
Meningococcal disease
Mumps
Novel influenza A virus infections
Pertussis
Plague
Poliomyelitis, paralytic
Poliovirus infection, nonparalytic
Psittacosis
Q fever
Rabies
Rubella
Salmonellosis
Severe acute respiratory syndrome (SARS-CoV)
Shiga toxin-producing (STEC)
Shigellosis
Smallpox
Spotted fever rickettsiosis
Streptococcal toxic-shock syndrome
Streptococcus pneumoniae, invasive disease
Syphilis
Tetanus
Toxic-shock syndrome (other than streptococcal)
Trichinellosis
Tuberculosis
Tularemia
Typhoid fever
Vancomycin infection
Varicella
Vibriosis
Viral hemorrhagic fevers
Yellow fever

Source: Centers for Disease Control and Prevention

Occupational Injury and Illness Classification

Another example of morbidity for which a classification system is required is injuries. There are different injury classification systems with applications in various settings. The Occupational Injury and Illness Classification System (OIICS) manual developed by the Bureau of Labor Statistics within the US Department of Labor outlines the classification system for coding the case characteristics of injuries, illnesses, and fatalities employed in the Survey of Occupational Injuries and Illnesses (SOII) and the Census of Fatal Occupational Injuries (CFOI) programs. This manual contains the rules of selection, code descriptions, code titles, and indices for data collection based on the nature of the injury or illness, the part of body affected, the primary (and secondary) source of injury or illness, and the event or exposure that led to the injury or illness. The OIICS was originally developed and released in 1992. Clarifications and corrections were incorporated into the manual in 2007. Exhibit 3.6 lists the different divisions addressed by the OIICS.

The Nature of Injury or Illness code structure is the most relevant for understanding disability patterns and is arranged so that traumatic injuries and disorders are listed first (in Division 1) while diseases are listed in Divisions 2–6. Exhibit 3.6 lists the divisions into which injuries and illnesses are arranged. Exhibit 3.7 presents a section of the coding system that has been extracted from the manual.

Exhibit 3.6: Divisions Used for Classifying Occupational Injuries and Illnesses

Division	Title
1	Traumatic injuries and disorders
2	Systemic diseases and disorders
3	Infectious and parasitic diseases
4	Neoplasms, tumors, and cancers
5	Symptoms, signs, and ill-defined conditions
6	Other diseases, conditions, and disorders
7	Exposures to disease—no illness incurred
8	Multiple diseases, conditions, and disorders
9999	Nonclassifiable

Exhibit 3.7: Coding System for Traumatic Injuries and Disorders (Division 1)

Code	Title
10	Traumatic injuries and disorders, unspecified
11	Traumatic injuries to bones, nerves, spinal cord
110	Traumatic injuries to bones, nerves, spinal cord, unspecified

(continued)

Exhibit 3.7 (continued)

Code	Title
111	Fractures
112	Traumatic injuries to spinal cord
1120	Traumatic injuries to spinal cord, unspecified
1121	Paralysis, paraplegia, quadriplegia
1129	Traumatic injuries to spinal cord, n.e.c.
113	Traumatic injuries to nerves, except the spinal cord
1130	Traumatic injuries to nerves, except the spinal cord, unspecified
1131	Pinched nerve
1139	Traumatic injuries to nerves, except the spinal cord, n.e.c.
118	Multiple traumatic injuries to bones, nerves, spinal cord
119	Traumatic injuries to bones, nerves, spinal cord, n.e.c.
12	Traumatic injuries to muscles, tendons, ligaments, joints, etc.
120	Traumatic injuries to muscles, tendons, ligaments, joints, etc., unspecified
121	Dislocations
1210	Dislocations, unspecified
1211	Herniated disks
1212	Dislocation of joints
1218	Multiple types of dislocations
1219	Dislocations, n.e.c.
122	Cartilage fractures and tears
1220	Cartilage fractures and tears, unspecified
1221	Meniscus tears
1229	Cartilage fractures and tears, n.e.c.
123	Sprains, strains, tears 1230 Sprains, strains, tears, unspecified
1231	Major tears to muscles, tendons, ligaments
1232	Sprains
1233	Strains
1238	Multiple sprains, strains, tears

Note: *n.e.c.* not elsewhere classified

Disability Classification

"Disability" is a condition that is hard to define and it does not lend itself to easy classification. A number of different classification systems have been developed and each has its own particular purpose. Care should taken when comparing the estimates from various sources because of differences in the criteria used to define disability. In the US, development of classification systems has been spurred by the needs of social insurance programs such as workmen's compensation, veterans' benefits, and Social Security.

Despite their widespread use each of the classification systems suffers from limitations of one kind or another. From a research perspective, the use of self-reported disability measures raises questions concerning the standardization of the participants' answers. Disability measures have also been problematic as public policy-making tools. The nation's social security insurance programs rely on the narrowly defined criteria of the disease model to determine disability. They do not adequately address psychological difficulties nor do they provide insight into certain social contributions to disability. Systems measuring limitations in major activities, on the other hand, may indicate the presence of some social contributions to disability but do not provide sufficient information to inform health interventions. These limitations have been recognized, but there has been limited success in developing a system that provides a sufficiently broad understanding of disability. Examples of disability classification systems are presented below.

International Classification of Impairments, Disabilities, and Handicaps

The WHO system categorizes a wide range of disabilities resulting from disease. The form and organization of the system are similar to WHO's *International Classification of Diseases* (ICD-9) especially in many of its subcategories; the overall structure, however, is informed by a theory of "planes of experience" in the development of illness and disability. This gives rise to four main categories: disease/disorder, impairment, disability, and handicap. The WHO manual describes these planes of experience as follows:

1. Something abnormal occurs within the individual; this may be present at birth or acquired later. A chain of causal circumstances, the "etiology," gives rise to changes in the structure or functioning of the body, the "pathology." These features are reflective of the medical model of disease.
2. Someone becomes aware of such an occurrence, and the pathological state is *exteriorized*. Most often the individual himself becomes aware of disease manifestations, usually referred to as "clinical disease." In behavioral terms, the individual has become or been made aware that he is unhealthy.
3. The performance or behavior of the individual may be altered as a result of this awareness, either consequentially or cognitively. Common activities may become restricted, and in this way the experience is *objectified*. Also relevant are psychological responses to the presence of disease. These experiences represent "disabilities," which reflect the consequences of impairments in terms of functional performance and activity by the individual.
4. Either the awareness itself, or the altered behavior or performance to which this gives rise, may place the individual at a disadvantage relative to others, thus *socializing* the experience. This plane reflects the response of society to the individual's experience, or to the extent to which the condition is a "handicap."

Unfortunately, this well-thought-out classification system for disabilities does not lend itself to a quantification of disabilities useful for our purposes. It is not commonly used as a framework for examining disability patterns in the US despite its many positive attributes.

International Classification of Functioning, Disability, and Health

The International Classification of Functioning, Disability, and Health (ICF) was developed by the World Health Organization and released in 2001. The ICF attempts to bridge many of these definitions by considering disability as an umbrella term for impairments, activity limitations, and participation restrictions. Rather than a dichotomous concept, disability is a gradient on which every person functions at different levels due to personal and environmental factors. While the ICF provides a common language for discussion of the concepts associated with disability, operationalizing this framework for survey questionnaires remains a challenge. Surveys must contain questions about a finite set of activities and set thresholds for levels of functioning over time. Exhibit 3.8 presents categories of disability utilized by the ICF.

Parts of this system have been adapted for use with federal surveys. In its supplemental questionnaires on adult and child functional limitations, the Survey of Income and Program Participation (SIPP) contains questions about whether respondents had difficulty performing a specific set of functional and participatory activities. For many activities, if a respondent reported difficulty, a follow-up question was asked to determine the severity of the limitation. Using these responses and others to questions about specific conditions and symptoms, this report presents disability as severe and nonsevere. These two measures combine to provide an overall estimate of disability prevalence.

Exhibit 3.8: Definition of Disability in the Communicative, Mental, and Physical Domains

The International Classification of Functioning, Disability and Health (ICF) categorizes types of disabilities into communicative, physical, and mental domains according to the criteria described below. While the characteristics of individuals with disabilities in a domain may be heterogeneous, the domains may group individuals with some common experiences. Because people can have more than one type of disability, they too may be identified as having disabilities in multiple domains. Disability among children less than 15 years old are not categorized into one of the three domains. Furthermore, it is possible for adults to have a disability for which the domain is not identified

People who have disability in the *communicative domain* reported one or more of the following:

1. Was blind or had difficulty seeing

(continued)

Exhibit 3.8 (continued)

2.Was deaf or had difficulty hearing
3.Had difficulty having their speech understood
People who have disability in the *physical domain* reported one or more of the following:
1.Used a wheelchair, cane, crutches, or walker
2.Had difficulty walking a quarter of a mile, climbing a flight of stairs, lifting something as heavy as a 10-lb bag of groceries, grasping objects, or getting in or out of bed
3.Listed arthritis or rheumatism, back or spine problem, broken bone or fracture, cancer, cerebral palsy, diabetes, epilepsy, head or spinal cord injury, heart trouble or atherosclerosis, hernia or rupture, high blood pressure, kidney problems, lung or respiratory problem, missing limbs, paralysis, stiffness or deformity of limbs, stomach/digestive problems, stroke, thyroid problem, or tumor/cyst/growth as a condition contributing to a reported activity limitation
People who have disability in the *mental domain* reported one or more of the following:
1.Had a learning disability, an intellectual disability, developmental disability or Alzheimer's disease, senility, or dementia
2.Had some other mental or emotional condition that seriously interfered with everyday activities

Workers' Compensation Disability Classifications

Established by the US Department of Labor, the federal Workers' Compensation program in cooperation with the various states and employers provides compensation as appropriate to workers injured or stricken ill on the job or as a result of a job. An injured worker's healthcare provider determines the extent of the disability. Cash benefits are directly related to the following disability classifications:

Temporary Total Disability: The injured worker's wage-earning capacity is lost totally, but only on a temporary basis.

Temporary Partial Disability: The wage-earning capacity is lost only partially, and on a temporary basis.

Permanent Total Disability: The employee's wage-earning capacity is permanently and totally lost. There is no limit on the number of weeks payable. In certain instances, an employee may continue to engage in business or employment, if his/her wages, combined with the weekly benefit, do not exceed the maximums set by law.

Permanent Partial Disability: Part of the employee's wage-earning capacity has been permanently lost on the job. If the work-related accident or date of disablement occurred before March 13, 2007, benefits are payable as long as the partial disability exists and results in wage loss. If there is no wage loss or reduced earnings as a result of the partial disability, only medical benefits are payable.

In addition, there is a special category (Schedule Loss) of Permanent Partial Disability, and involves loss of eyesight or hearing, or loss of a part of the body or its use. Compensation is limited to a certain number of weeks, according to a schedule set by law.

Disfigurement: Serious and permanent disfigurement to the face, head, or neck may entitle the worker to compensation up to a maximum of $20000, depending upon the date of the accident.

Census Bureau/ACS Disability Classification

The Census Bureau currently collects data on disability through the American Community Survey (ACS). The questions in the current ACS questionnaires cover six disability types:

- Hearing difficulty: Deaf or having serious difficulty hearing
- Vision difficulty: Blind or having serious difficulty seeing, even when wearing glasses
- Cognitive difficulty: Having difficulty remembering, concentrating, or making decisions because of a physical, mental, or emotional problem
- Ambulatory difficulty: Having serious difficulty walking or climbing stairs
- Self-care difficulty: Having difficulty bathing or dressing
- Independent living difficulty: Because of a physical, mental, or emotional problem, having difficulty doing errands alone such as visiting a doctor's office or shopping

Respondents who report any one of the six disability types are considered to have a disability. The Census Bureau pools together 12-months of data collection to produce annual estimates for geographies with populations of 65000 or more. With a 36-month period of data collection, a three-year estimate is produced. In 2013, the first 5-year estimates (pooling 60 months of data collection) on the disability status of individuals were produced for all geographies including census tracts and block groups.

ACS reports present the number of residents with a (i.e., any) disability and breaks these down into the age groups of under 18 years, 18–64 years, and 65 years and older. More detailed statistics are presented on disability related to the labor force. The disability status of those in the labor force and employed, those in the labor force and unemployed, and those not in the force is broken down into the six categories listed above. Data are also presented on the disabled in relation to their poverty status.

Childhood Disability Classification

In order to address the needs of school-age children affected by disabilities, the Individuals with Disabilities in Education Act (IDEA) was passed in 2004. The IDEA's disability terms and definitions guide how States define disability and determine who is eligible for free appropriate public education under the special education law. In order to fully meet the definition (and eligibility for special education and related services) as a "child with a disability," a child's educational performance must be adversely affected due to the disability. The following conditions are considered disabilities according to IDEA criteria:

- Autism
- Deaf-blindness
- Deafness
- Developmental delay
- Emotional disturbance
- Hearing impairment
- Intellectual disability
- Multiple disabilities
- Orthopedic impairment
- Other health impairment
- Specific learning disability
- Speech or language impairment
- Traumatic brain injury
- Visual impairment including blindness

The federal government has established a database for accessing state-level data about school-aged children with disabilities (ages 3–21) served under the Individuals with Disabilities Education Act. These data can be accessed through the www.data. gov website.

The Classification of Mental Illness

The classification of morbidity related to mental problems is conceptualized somewhat differently from physical illness, and this is reflected in a classification system specific to mental disorders. Mental illness involves disorders of mood, behavior, or thought processes. This sets this category of health problems apart from physical disorders; differences in etiology, symptomatology, progression, diagnostic procedures, and treatment modalities are clearly distinguished. The fact that mental disorders are generally not subject to clinical diagnostic procedures has important implications for the classification system that has evolved.

The definitive reference on the classification of mental disorder is the *Diagnostic and Statistical Manual of Mental Disorders* (American Psychiatric Association 2013). Now in its fifth edition, it is commonly referred to as DSM-V. Its 16 major categories of mental illness and over 300 identified mental conditions are exhaustive. The DSM classification system is derived in part from the ICD system discussed earlier. It is essentially structured in the same manner, with a five-digit code being utilized. The fourth digit indicates the variety of the particular disorder under discussion, and the fifth digit refers to any special considerations related to the case. The nature of the fifth-digit modifier varies depending on the disorder under consideration. (Exhibits 3.9 and 3.10 indicate the major classifications within DSM-V and present a representative sampling of the coding of mental disorders.) Unlike the other classification systems discussed, the DSM system contains rather detailed descriptions of the disorders categorized therein.

Exhibit 3.9: Diagnostic Categories Utilized in the Diagnostic and Statistical Manual of Mental Disorders (Fourth Edition) (DSM-V)

Category	Example
Neurodevelopmental disorders	Mental retardation
Schizophrenia spectrum and other psychotic disorders	Schizophrenia
Bipolar and related disorders	Manic-depressive disorder
Depressive disorders	Depression
Anxiety disorders	Generalized anxiety disorder
Obsessive-compulsive and related disorders	Obsessive-compulsive disorder
Trauma- and stressor-related disorders	Posttraumatic stress disorder
Dissociative disorders	Amnesia
Somatic symptom disorders	Hypochondriasis
Feeding and eating disorders	Bulimia
Elimination disorders	Urinary tract symptoms
Sleep-wake disorders	Insomnia
Sexual dysfunctions	Male erectile disorder
Gender dysphoria	Gender identity disorder
Disruptive, impulse control, and conduct disorders	Kleptomania
Substance use and addictive disorders	Drug use disorder
Neurocognitive disorders	Dementia
Personality disorders	Sociopathy
Paraphilic disorders	Pedophilia
Other disorders	

It may be worthwhile to present another conceptualization of the categories of mental disorder that is more straightforward (oversimplified, some might say), but is both more useful for general discussions of mental illness and more in keeping with popular conceptualizations of mental disorders. The significance of the various categories for the contemporary healthcare delivery system will be noted as each is discussed.

This system begins by distinguishing between *organic* and *nonorganic mental disorders*. Only a small fraction (approximately 5 %) of mental disorders fall into the organic category, and many would classify these as physical illnesses because of the presence of brain damage, neurological dysfunction, or chemical imbalance. The small proportion of cases is noteworthy, since they require almost total care and the significance of this category is expected to increase as victims of Alzheimer's disease become more numerous. Brain-damaged patients generally do not benefit from active medical intervention and are typically cared for in custodial-type institutions.

Exhibit 3.10: Representative Examples of DSM-V Codes for Mental Disorders

Panic disorders
300.21—panic disorder with agoraphobia
300.22—agoraphobia without history of panic disorder
300.01—panic disorder without agoraphobia
Generalized anxiety
300—anxiety disorder NOS
300.02—generalized anxiety disorder
Phobias
300.23—social phobia
300.29—specific phobia
Obsessive-compulsive disorder
300.3—obsessive-compulsive disorder

The remainder of disorders are nonorganic, or *functional*. They are termed functional disorders because their common characteristic is interference with social role performance and interpersonal relationships. Unlike the organic disorders, functional disorders typically do not have an identifiable underlying biological basis, and in fact their etiology is generally not known. These conditions are manifested primarily by disorders of mood, thought processes, and behavior.

Functional disorders are commonly divided into three major categories: neuroses, psychoses, and personality disorders. *Neuroses* include the relatively mild disorders that are generally associated with low intensity care (e.g., psychological counseling) and include such conditions as anxiety, compulsiveness, and various "nervous" conditions. These are conditions that typically affect only one dimension of a person's being; the remaining aspects of personality are essentially normal. These disorders are virtually always cared for on an outpatient basis and have limited significance for the formal healthcare system.

Psychoses are often thought of as more serious forms of neuroses, although many contend that there is a qualitative difference between the two. Psychotic conditions are often extreme in their manifestations and tend to disorder completely the lives of the individuals so affected. This category includes schizophrenia, depression, and extreme paranoia—conditions that often require institutionalization in mental hospitals since they are usually too severe and disruptive to be treated in a general hospital setting. These are the conditions that often entail psychotropic drug therapy, electroconvulsive shock treatment, and at times psychosurgery

The final category, *personality disorders*, represents something of a residual category. It includes a variety of conditions that do not fit neatly into the other categories. Included are such disorders as antisocial behavior, sexual deviance, and alcohol and drug abuse. The contents of this category exhibit the most variety, since this is the "bucket" in which newly diagnosed or redefined conditions often end up. Other examples included in this category are homosexuality, eating disorders, and child abuse, all conditions that at some time in the recent past would not have been considered medical conditions. Although these disparate conditions are hard to categorize, they could be said to share the characteristics of unpredictability, unclear etiology, and unresponsiveness to any type of therapy other than behavior-modification techniques. Personality disorders are of growing significance for the healthcare delivery system in that certain of them are receiving inordinate attention at this point in time; examples of these include substance abuse and eating disorders.

While this system is useful for understanding the nature of mental disorder within a population, limited data are collected using these categories. As a practical matter, the technical classification system represented by DSM guidelines is more commonly used in psychiatric epidemiology.

Cause of Death Classification

Some mention should be made of the manner in which death is classified. A cause of death is assigned to each deceased individual and registered through the standard death certificate that is used throughout the US. To the extent that cause of death can be considered as something of a proxy for morbidity, basic information on the assignment of cause of death may be informative. Historically, there was a fairly close correlation between common maladies and common causes of death. The immediate cause of death was typically the primary cause of death, with few complicating factors involved. That connection can still be made today to a certain extent, in that the leading causes of death (heart disease and cancer) reflect common maladies within the population.

Contemporary population scientists place less emphasis on mortality analysis than they did in the past. In the US, the mortality rate has dropped to the point that death is a relatively rare event. As a component of population change, mortality has become less important than fertility and both have become less important than migration. Further, the correspondence between mortality and morbidity has become diminished. Because of the preponderance of chronic disease within the US population, death certificates are less and less likely to capture the underlying disease. Chronic diseases typically do not kill people, but those affected typically die from some complication (of diabetes, AIDS or cancer, for example). This is not to say that mortality analysis cannot provide insights into morbidity patterns, but that the situation is much more complicated than in the past, and analysts require a better understanding of disease processes (and the vagaries of death certificates) today.

The *causes of death* affecting a population are a major factor in determining the level of mortality. Populations in different times and places are subject to different causes of death. Knowing the number of people who died is one thing, but knowing what they died from provides valuable insights into the overall health status of the population and the types of health conditions that afflict that population. Information on cause of death in the US is compiled from certificates filed with health authorities on the occasion of any death. Since virtually every death is accompanied by a death certificate, the information on cause of death is fairly complete. However, given today's morbidity patterns, it is increasingly difficult to specify the ultimate cause of death. With a preponderance of chronic diseases, it is often the case that death can and should be attributed to a factor other than the proximate cause of death. For example, patients with AIDS do not typically die as a direct result of AIDS but due to system failure caused by AIDS. Similarly, individuals affected by diabetes are often said to die from "complications of diabetes." While the immediate cause of death may be kidney failure, it is useful to know that diabetes was the underlying cause. Similarly, obesity, while not an immediate cause of death, is increasingly being listed as a contributing factor. While the death certificate provides space for the recording of contributing conditions, the complexity of chronic disease may make it difficult to determine the exact cause of death.

While death certificates represent a significant source of data for mortality analysis, there are issues that require caution in their use. There is not universal agreement as to the determination of which factor is the immediate cause of death. There are, in fact, differences that exist from community to community with regard to the classification of contributing and proximate factors. There may also be a tendency, hopefully not widespread, to misrepresent the cause of death for various reasons. There may be reluctance, for example, to specify AIDS or some other sexually transmitted disease as a cause of death. Similarly, there may be reticence with regard to specifying alcohol- or drug-related conditions as the cause of death. The slippage with regard to accurate classification of cause of death is also exacerbated due to the trend toward employment of coroners who are not physicians. In fact, in some jurisdictions, the coroner may be an elected office. For these reasons, it is important to use mortality data with caution and certainly to consider the full variety of contributors to mortality.

In the US, the International Classification of Disease classification system is used to assign cause of death. The tenth version of the ICD system is slowly being adapted but most US healthcare organizations are still using the nineth version (ICD-9). Exhibits 3.1 and 3.2 above provide information on the ICD classification system used for both applying a diagnosis to a live patient as well as assigning a cause of death to a deceased individual.

References

Advance Healthcare Network. (2015). An inpatient prospective payment system refresher: MS-DRGs. Retrieved from http://health-information.advanceweb.com/Web-Extras/CCS-Prep/An-Inpatient-Prospective-Payment-System-Refresher-MS-DRGs-2.aspx.

American Psychiatric Association. (2013). *Diagnostic and statistical manual V*. Arlington, VA: American Psychiatric Publishing.

Centers for Disease Control and Prevention. (2014). Summary of notifiable diseases—United States, 2014. *Morbidity Mortality Weekly Report, 61*(53), 1–122.

Centers for Disease Control and Prevention. (2015). International classification of diseases, ninth revision, clinical modification (ICD-9-CM). Retrieved from http://www.cdc.gov/nchs/icd/icd9cm.htm.

Additional Resources

American Psychological Association. (2013). *Diagnostic and statistical manual IV.*
National Research Council Publication. *The aging population in the twenty-first century: Statistics for health policy.* Retrieved from www.cdc.gov (notifiable diseases; disease registries).
www.cdc.gov/nchs (Incidence/prevalence data).
www.census.gov (American Community Survey).
www.cms.gov (Diagnostic related groups).
www.data.gov (IDEA statistics).
www.dol.gov/dol/topic/workcomp/ (Workers compensation).
www.who.org (International Classification of Impairments, Disabilities, and Handicaps; International Classification of Functioning, Disability, and Health).
wwwn.cdc.gov/oiics/ (Occupational Illness and Injury Classification System).

Chapter 4
Identifying Morbidity

Introduction

The primary purpose of the study of morbidity is to determine the level of sickness and disability exhibited by a population. Having previously defined morbidity, the challenge becomes one of identifying morbid conditions and calculating the level of morbidity within the population based on that information. There are a number of ways in which morbid conditions can be identified and no single method adequately serves this purpose. The use of a variety of methods is required in the US because there is no centralized registry of morbid conditions nor any systematic process for the comprehensive collection of morbidity data. While data on fertility and mortality are virtually 100 % complete for the US population due to the mandated use of standardized birth and death certificates, no such process is in place for the reporting of incidents of ill-health.

The lack of a centralized repository of data is something of a moot point in that the available data capture systems for morbid conditions are limited in their usefulness. With a few exceptions, there are limited opportunities for the electronic capture and/or reporting of identified cases of disease. Although the Centers for Disease Control and Prevention (CDC) has introduced the technological capability for the reporting of selected health conditions, there are no such mechanisms available for the majority of health problems. The primary generators of data on morbid conditions—healthcare providers—do not participate in any systematic process of data compilation.

© Springer New York 2016
R.K. Thomas, *In Sickness and In Health*, Applied Demography Series 6,
DOI 10.1007/978-1-4939-3423-2_4

Even if there was a central repository and all relevant parties had access to efficient means of reporting morbid cases, the actual reporting of cases would still be limited. While the reporting of certain conditions (e.g., HIV/AIDS, tuberculosis) is required by law, there is no mechanism for enforcing these requirements on the hundreds of thousands of healthcare providers and healthcare organizations that might encounter these cases. For certain types of health conditions it is felt that the reporting is fairly complete—that is, most cases are actually reported to the appropriate authorities. However, for the majority of conditions it is felt that a significant—and often unknown—level of underreporting exists.

Beyond limitations in the reporting of data on morbidity, the usefulness of data on cases that are actually identified is limited due to the variations that exist in diagnosing health conditions. The variation that exists among causes of death, for example, has been clearly documented, so, to the extent that death records might be considered as a proxy for morbidity, the discrepancies that exists in this regard makes the use of death data as an indicator of morbidity status highly questionable.

This subjective aspect of diagnosis is not limited to cause of death, however. While the medical profession establishes agreed-upon guidelines for what constitutes a "case," issues remain with regard to the establishment of a diagnosis. Thresholds for the specification of a disease are established based on the best available evidence supported by professional consensus (although this may be difficult to reach in some cases). For example, the level of blood pressure that constitutes a diagnosis of "high blood pressure" or the body mass index level that indicates "obesity" are established based on current knowledge. These are not absolute indicators but represent best estimates of when a non-case is redefined as a case. Because of their somewhat arbitrary nature, such standards are prone to change over time and sometimes in response to factors other than advances in medical science. To a certain extent, the diagnosis of disease is as much an art as a science, and this often leads to wide variations in the diagnosis of conditions from one practitioner to another or from one community to another.

The indications for a particular health condition may change over time. Longstanding conditions (e.g., menopause) may subsequently be deemed to be clinically relevant while others (e.g., homosexuality) may be clinically declassified (and, thus, no longer be counted for morbidity purposes). In addition, the criteria or threshold for identification of a condition may change over time, as in the case of hypertension (high blood pressure) in which the threshold has steadily been lowered in recent years. Further, the classification of a condition as a "disease" may reflect the availability of a treatment rather than a thoughtful reconsideration of the nature of the condition.

Underlying each of these issues is the special case of "personal health data." Personal health data are unique in that, unlike virtually every other type of personal data, they are protected by virtue of professional ethics backed up by fairly stringent legal protections. While the simple reporting of a case does not in itself represent a violation of any privacy standard, the reporting of a case that includes any information that would make the patient identifiable is clearly prohibited. Thus, the demographic attributes that would be useful in gaining an understanding of the conditions surrounding the case can only be specified under very carefully controlled circumstances. To report a case for a married 40-year-old African-American female living in ZIP Code 12345 in such-and-such state would be considered a breach of confidentiality on the grounds that it might be possible to identify that person. There is particular sensitivity with regard to the release of data that might present the individual in an unfavorable light, e.g., a diagnosis of HIV, schizophrenia, or drug addiction. While most personal health data is innocuous and would not represent any sort of threat if revealed, the possibility of misuse of these data has led to the enactment of stringent controls.

That point leads to the last consideration. While there is some benefit to simply identifying and counting a case of a particular health condition, that information is of limited usefulness without additional data. For most purposes for which morbidity data would be used, it is important to be able to determine the location of the event (e.g., an accident) and/or the residence of the affected individual. Further, it is important to understand other, mostly demographic, attributes of the affected individual. For almost every purpose, it is important to know the age, sex, and race of the individual and, for most purposes for which the data will be used, marital status, living arrangements, education, income level, occupation and even religious affiliation are likely to be useful. The availability of this supplementary information varies widely depending on the source of the data and the manner in which cases are reported. Unfortunately, this information is lacking in most cases.

Identifying Morbidity

The basis for all epidemiological analysis is the determination of the types and levels of morbidity, disability, and mortality characterizing a particular population. The denominator in this equation—the population at risk—is usually readily available. The problematic aspect of the equation is the numerator—that is, the existing number of cases of the condition. As a consequence, much of the research that takes place with regard to disease incidence/prevalence focuses on identifying the number and characteristics of the cases of the health condition under consideration.

Our existing knowledge of the morbidity characteristics of the US population is based on a variety of sources. "Cases"—that is, incidents of ill-health—are officially identified in clinical settings, and this is the primary source of reported cases of morbid conditions. These cases may ultimately be included in disease registries of various types. However, incidents of ill-health are only relevant if they have been identified by the "system." Clearly, there are large numbers of cases of ill-health that are not identified and thus not reported.

In clinical settings a diagnosis is made by a health professional, usually a physician and usually based on the results of diagnostic tests. These diagnoses, which provide the basis for identifying the morbidity characterizing a population, can be recorded at a physician office, a clinic, an outpatient diagnostic facility, or a hospital, often based on the results of tests performed by an external laboratory. A primary diagnosis is typically attached to the individual based on presenting symptoms. This process may involve a preliminary diagnosis (e.g., upon arrival at the hospital emergency department) which will be converted to a "final" diagnosis upon discharge from treatment. The challenge for the diagnostician is to sort through various symptoms to determine from among the many options the correct diagnosis or diagnoses. This process involves "differential diagnosis" in which the diagnostician seeks to systemically eliminate unlikely diagnoses until an ultimate determination can be made.

It is not unusual for an individual presenting for treatment to have more than one health condition and, thus, multiple diagnoses (or the presence of "comorbidity"). The primary diagnosis may be referred to as the "first-listed" diagnosis in a medical record. Any comorbidity would be considered a secondary diagnosis and listed as such on the medical record. In calculating the amount of morbidity characterizing a population, analysts may consider either the first-listed diagnoses or any-listed diagnosis, depending on their objectives (Senathirajah et al. 2011). Obviously, counting all diagnoses will yield a much larger number of conditions (and certainly more conditions than there are patients) and a truer picture of the morbidity of the population than only using the first-listed diagnosis.

There may be cases in which an inaccurate diagnosis is recorded. Most incorrect diagnoses are accidental and reflect inconclusive test results or the inaccurate interpretation of these results (Kistler et al. 2010). There are occasions, thankfully rare, when an incorrect diagnosis may deliberately be assigned. This might occur when the practitioner is seeking to protect the patient, the patient's family, or some other party from embarrassment or liability. The misidentification of a case may be made when a case is diagnosed or at the point where the diagnosis is entered into an official record. There have been incidences in which celebrities, for example, when hospitalized were assigned a misleading diagnosis in order to protect their privacy should their medical records be inappropriately accessed. This could also happen in the case of a family doctor who is loathe to assign a diagnosis of HIV or some mental disorder on the grounds that members of the family might be upset. Fortunately, such cases are thought to be extremely rare today.

There are also situations—and in this case all too common—in which an identified case is not reported. Given the large number of physicians and other practitioners, hospitals, medical laboratories, and other entities, it is not surprising that some cases that should be reported fall through the cracks. After all, despite the reporting of certain conditions being required by law, disease reporting still remains an essentially voluntary activity. The failure to report is usually unintentional as in the case of the harried physician who identifies an HIV-infected person among his patients but neglects to report the case to public health authorities. Again, there may be cases in which a practitioner deliberately fails to report a diagnosed case and for much the same reasons as above—fear that the identity of the affected party may become known.

An important consideration when it comes to case-finding is the fact that variations in the assignment of diagnoses to individuals may reflect demographic traits (Berger 2008). The tendency for clinicians to apply different diagnoses to individuals based on age, sex, or race is well documented. For example, symptoms of a heart attack may be interpreted differently for males and females, antisocial behavior may be attributed to one diagnosis in a teenager but to another in an adult, or obesity may be less likely to be diagnosed in an African-American woman than in a white woman exhibiting the same characteristics. Further, the demographic attributes of the *clinician* may be a factor in determining the diagnosis with, for example, an older white male physician interpreting a patient's symptoms differently from a younger African-American female physician.

The determination of the level of psychiatric morbidity represents a particular challenge. While a diagnosis of psychiatric morbidity is typically made by a psychiatrist or other clinician or by a technician under the supervision of a physician, there are relatively few diagnostics tests for use in identifying psychiatric disorders. Although a small portion of mental disorders can be attributed to some underlying biological pathology (e.g., nervous system damage), most mental conditions are thought to reflect either internal psychological pathology or the influence of external stressors. Neither of these lend themselves to traditional medical diagnostic techniques. Thus, cases are "found" primarily based on subjective judgment of the practitioner. Exhibit 4.1 describes the challenges involved in disease case-finding.

Exhibit 4.1: Challenges to Case-Finding

"Case-finding" refers to the various approaches utilized to identify incidents of ill-health within a population. In epidemiology, a case refers to an animal (in this context a human being) that has the specified disease or condition under investigation. In a more general sense, a case is any example of morbidity within a population. While many cases may be discovered through reports issued by various agencies, these reports may not adequately represent all of the people affected, and more aggressive case-finding may be required.

Epidemiologists have developed criteria for classifying a suspected disease case. A case that meets the clinical case definition but is not laboratory confirmed or epidemiologically linked to another probable or confirmed case is considered a *probable* case. A case that is laboratory confirmed or meets the clinical case definition and is epidemiologically linked to a confirmed or probable case is a *confirmed* case.

While targeted case-finding reflects efforts toward disease control in the case of an outbreak, public health authorities conduct routine and incident-specific morbidity and mortality surveillance using a variety of sources. These might include disease surveillance systems, vital statistics reports, hospital discharge abstracts, community surveys, disease registries, and active case-finding.

In examining a disease outbreak, investigators must determine the characteristics of the people who have contracted the disease, when they became

(continued)

Exhibit 4.1 (continued)

symptomatic, and where they may have been exposed. This information may help identify a potential exposure source and/or the cause of the outbreak. When attempting to find cases at the beginning of an outbreak, a wide net is typically cast. This allows for the determination of the size and geographic boundaries of the outbreak, since cases that are recognized first may represent only the "tip of the iceberg."

Cases can be identified through active or passive case-finding strategies. *Active* case-finding involves soliciting information from health facilities and laboratories to identify additional cases. Another method of active case-finding involves screening an exposed population using a diagnostic test. *Passive* case-finding, which is less aggressive and requires less resources, may involve examining county or state surveillance data to identify cases reported through the communicable disease reporting system. In an outbreak situation, some cases may be identified through passive case-finding, supplemented by active case-finding. Multiple sources may be used to find cases, and some situations may require creativity on the part of the investigator.

In searching for cases, physician offices, clinics, hospitals, and laboratories may be contacted for information. Emergency room records for all patients seen with the illness can be reviewed or specimens requested from clinicians for all patients who meet a clinical case definition. Infection control practitioners may be asked to review medical records of patients with a particular diagnosis. In some situations it may be appropriate to query the community through local television, radio, or newspapers, particularly if members of the public may be able to provide critical information (e.g., on a contaminated food product).

Investigators may look at records such as wedding invitation lists, guest books, credit card receipts, and customer lists maintained by establishments involved in an outbreak. Hospital intensive-care units, microbiology laboratories, medical examiners, veterinarians, and site investigations at locations visited by an identified case may be checked to determine the source of the patient's exposure. When exposure has occurred in a defined setting within a defined population, it may be effective to ask every person within the population about symptoms. For example, everyone who was at a church picnic, wedding, or school function or on a cruise ship may be queried.

Even with active case-finding, several factors make it difficult to identify or confirm all existing cases. Ultimately, multiple sources may be needed to find the targeted cases, and synthesis of data on the part of the investigator may be required. The issues in case-finding described above call for rigor on the part of those involved in the case-finding process as well as caution on the part of researchers who are interpreting the data.

Reported Cases

Most of what is known about the morbidity patterns of populations within the US is derived from reported cases of disease and disability. The reported cases approach to case-finding involves the identification of cases based on the formal recording of cases by healthcare organizations. The reporting of certain health conditions is required by law and these data are entered into a national data bank. Local health departments or individual healthcare institutions might also maintain registries for purposes of tracking cases. In other instances, the number of reported cases may be compiled through periodic surveys of the organizations that deal with a particular condition. For example, the National Center for Health Statistics (NCHS) might assemble data on all hospital discharges for a particular time period to determine the number of cases of a given condition treated within the nation's hospitals. Similarly, the Centers for Medicare and Medicaid Services might collect data from all providers of services to Medicare patients in order to determine the magnitude of a specific health problem.

Most cases are generated through interaction with the healthcare system. Through the routine activities of physician offices, clinics, hospitals, medical laboratories, and other healthcare organizations, patient diagnoses are recorded, and these ultimately represent the bulk of the reported cases of morbidity. Every year tens of millions physician office visits are logged along with millions of hospital admissions. Each episode generates at least one diagnosis and most of them more than one.

The reported cases method of case-finding has both advantages and disadvantages. With the computerization of many healthcare databases, the compilation of comprehensive data on a wide range of health problems is easier today than at any time in the past. A large volume of data is readily available, and an extensive amount of information useful for epidemiological studies is often accessible for reported cases. On the other hand, this method suffers to the extent that not all sources of care are included in the reporting and compilation of data, criteria for reporting and even defining conditions vary from area to area, and multiple reporting of the same case is always a possibility. As a result, underreporting is a problem with regard to many diseases, and further inquiry is necessary if these data are to be used. On the positive side, disease surveillance data as currently collected make possible analyses at the individual, group (e.g., age cohort), and geographic levels.

The major drawback to using reported cases as the basis for the numerator, however, is inherent in the process itself. Reported cases are just that—cases that have been both diagnosed and entered into an appropriate data bank. Many cases are never diagnosed, especially for such conditions as mental disorders (for which much subjectivity is involved in the diagnostic process). In fact, the "known" cases of many diseases represent only the tip of the iceberg. For some conditions, more cases may go undetected than detected. Further, reporting is less than complete and is often selective. Therefore, uncritical utilization of reported data can result in misleading conclusions (Kituse and Cicourel 1963).

Much of what we know about morbidity within the US population is based on data drawn from various registries of patients with health conditions. The CDC maintains a number of registries that track certain types of health problems. The National Notifiable Diseases Surveillance System (NNDSS), noted in Chap. 3, tracks the condition that must be reported to public health authorities. By 1990, all 50 states were using CDC's National Electronic Telecommunications System for Surveillance (NETSS) to report individual case data that included demographic information (without personal identifiers) for most nationally notifiable diseases. These data are important for evaluating the demographic correlates of the occurrence of infectious diseases, monitoring infectious disease morbidity trends, and determining the relative disease burden among demographically diverse subpopulations (Centers for Disease Control and Prevention 2013).

Potential (suspect) cases of notifiable diseases are reported to local, regional, or state public health authorities. These reports might be based on a positive laboratory test, clinical symptoms, or epidemiologic criteria. When a suspect case is determined to meet the national case definition, de-identified data are sent to the CDC. This can include information reported to public health by laboratories and healthcare providers, along with other information collected during public health investigations.

Currently, there are 52 infectious diseases designated as notifiable at the national level. Infectious disease data are also available for all 50 states, the District of Columbia, and 122 selected cities. The data are available on a monthly basis in *Morbidity and Mortality Weekly Report*, a CDC publication, and at http://www2. cdc.gov:81/mmwr/mmwr.htm. Additional information on notifiable diseases can be found at http://www.cdc.gov.

The CDC also maintains specialized registries focusing on specific diseases. One example would be the Outpatient Influenza-like Illness Surveillance Network (ILINet) consisting of about 2400 healthcare providers in 50 states reporting approximately 16 million patient visits each year. Each week, approximately 1300 outpatient care sites around the country report data to CDC on the total number of patients seen and the number of those patients with influenza-like illness (ILI). The percentage of patient visits to healthcare providers for ILI reported each week is weighted on the basis of state population and compared each week with the national baseline.

Another source of reported cases is through the abstraction of data from various repositories of patient records. The primary source of such data is the NCHS which has a number of such initiatives underway. This essentially involves identifying a sample of healthcare providers (e.g., physician offices, hospitals, nursing homes) and drawing a sample of their patient records from which data are abstracted. The key surveys that generate data related to morbidity are the National Ambulatory Medical Care Survey (NAMCS), the National Hospital Discharge Survey (NHDS), and the National Hospital Ambulatory Medical Care Survey (NHAMCS). The NAMCS generates data on reasons for the physician visit, outpatient diagnoses, and outpatient procedures, as well as drugs prescribed. The NHDS abstracts data on reason for hospital admissions, diagnoses assigned, and procedures performed. The NHAMCS abstracts data related to the use of hospital-based ambulatory facilities such as the emergency department, outpatient diagnostics, and outpatient surgery. This survey generates data on reason for emergency department visit, ED diagnoses and procedures, and outpatient surgeries performed. The NHDS was last conducted in 2010 and has been supplanted by the National Hospital Care Survey (NHCS). The NHCS merges the former NHDS with the NHAMCS to create a new survey form that covers inpatient care, emergency services, hospital outpatient services, and hospital-provided ambulatory care surgery. Exhibit 4.2 presents information on surveys conducted by the NCHS.

To the extent that mortality data are used as a proxy for morbidity data, the available information on the US population is of very high quality. The pervasive use of mortality data, however, is probably more a function of its ready availability and its ease of interpretation than of its current relevance as a morbidity indicator. The crude mortality rate is the least refined of the various measures of morbidity and, unless it is adjusted to account for interpopulation variations in demographic, socioeconomic, and healthcare utilization characteristics, reliance on the crude death rate as a proxy for morbidity can generate misleading conclusions. Further, the fact that the measure uses the total population as its denominator masks a great deal of subgroup differences.

An examination of the causes of death for a population provides more meaningful insights into the morbidity patterns than the overall mortality rate. An overall mortality rate of 10 deaths per 1000 residents is an aggregate figure that combines the death rates for a wide variety of causes. Thus, the rate of 10 may be the end result of 3 persons per 1000 dying from heart disease, two from cancer, and two from stroke. The remainder of the 10/1000 rate reflects the aggregate mortality for hundreds of other causes of death. The emphasis on specific causes of death reflects the notion that some causes of death may be more important than others as a reflection of population morbidity. The use of cause-specific data also makes comparisons between populations more meaningful.

One other frequently utilized mortality indicator is the infant mortality rate, and this is sometimes considered a proxy for a population's overall health status. Although this measure only applies to a limited segment of the population (i.e., those under 1 year of age), it is considered by many as more useful than the overall mortality rate. The premise is that the infant mortality rate is much more than an outcome measure for the healthcare system. Rather, the level of infant mortality is a function of environmental safety, diet, prenatal care, the educational and economic status of the parents, the age of the mother, the occurrence of neglect and abuse, and a number of other factors. Thus, infant mortality is thought to reflect the combined impact of multiple contributors to health and well-being. As with the overall mortality rate, however, infant deaths occur rarely enough that measures of infant mortality have less salience as indicators of a population's health than they did historically.

The NCHS maintains a registry of all deaths occurring within the US. This registry is compiled from death certificates filed at the local level (i.e., county health department) which are batched for each state and forwarded to NCHS for processing and analysis. The data collected on the standard death certificate include primary cause of death, contributing causes, and individual demographic and socioeconomic characteristics such as sex, race, ethnicity, last occupation, place of residence, and place of death. Using these data, demographers can begin to study the relationship between the cause of death and a variety of demographic variables. The association between cause of death and certain demographic attributes provides insights into observed morbidity patterns.

The NCHS does not field any surveys devoted to mental health epidemiology. However, through the National Ambulatory Medical Care Survey and the NHDS, the NCHS collects a considerable amount of data related to the use of mental health services. The former tallies the various mental health conditions for which patients present themselves at the physician office; the latter enumerates the number of hospital discharges that are associated with a mental health diagnosis. Data collected through these surveys of healthcare providers represent the only available information on reported cases of psychiatric morbidity.

Exhibit 4.2: The National Center for Health Statistics

The NCHS is considered by many to be the Census Bureau of healthcare. As a division of the CDC, the NCHS performs a number of invaluable functions related to data on health and healthcare. Since 1960, the Center has carried out the tasks of data collection and analysis, data dissemination, and the development of methodologies for research on health issues. The NCHS also coordinates the various state centers for health statistics.

The compilation and analysis of data on morbidity is an important function, and the Center has been responsible for the development of much of the epidemiologic data available. To this end, a variety of registries are maintained on health-related topics, some in conjunction with the CDC. A major responsibility is the compilation, analysis, and publication of vital statistics for the US and each relevant subarea. This massive task of compiling and analyzing births and deaths provides the basis for the calculation of fertility and mortality rates. These statistics, in turn, provide the basis for various health-related estimates and projections made by other organizations.

In addition to the data compiled from various registration sources, the center is the foremost administrator of healthcare surveys in the nation. Its sample surveys are generally large scale and fall into two categories: community-based surveys and facility-based surveys. The National Health Interview Survey (NHIS), in which data are collected annually from approximately 50000 households, is perhaps the center's most important survey. The NHIS is the nation's primary source of data on the incidence/prevalence of health conditions, health status, the injuries and disabilities characterizing the population, health services utilization, and a variety of other health-related topics. Other surveys that involve a sample from the community are the National Medical Care Utilization and Expenditures Survey (NMCUES), the National Health and Nutrition Examination Survey (NHANES), and the National

---

(continued)

Exhibit 4.2 (continued)

Survey of Family Growth (NSFG). Another survey, the National Maternal and Infant Health Survey (NMIHS), involves a sampling of certificates of birth, fetal death, and infant death.

The NCHS also surveys a variety of healthcare institutions in its efforts to identify morbidity levels (among other objectives). Data are abstracted from the records of physician offices, hospitals and nursing homes. Healthcare providers are randomly selected for participation in the data collection process. The NAMCS samples the patient records of 2500 office-based physicians to obtain data on diagnoses, treatment, and medications prescribed, along with information on the characteristics of both physicians and patients. Important facility-based surveys include the NHDS and the National Nursing Home Survey (NNHS).

Historically, the NCHS collected data on hospital utilization via the NHDS. The NHDS was last conducted in 2010 and has been supplanted by the NHCS. The NHCS merges the former NHDS with the NHAMCS to create a new survey form that covers inpatient care, emergency services, hospital outpatient services, and hospital-provided ambulatory care surgery. Data are abstracted from a sample of medical records for patients who are hospitalized or use hospital outpatient services. The NHCS reports include personal health data to allow for tracking patients across the various services.

Additional surveys conducted by the Center include the National Survey of Ambulatory Surgery (NSAS), the National Nursing Home Survey (NNHS), the National Home and Hospice Care Survey (NHHCS), the National Study of Long-Term Care Providers (NSLTCP), and the National Survey of Residential Care Facilities (NSRCF). These surveys vary in their frequency of administration.

The data collected through NCHS programs are disseminated in a variety of ways. The Center's resources include annual publications such as *Health, United States* (the "official" government compendium of statistics on the nation's health) and a series of publications such as *Vital and Health Statistics*. Much of the data collected—including raw data from NCHS surveys—is available online from the NCHS website. The NCHS also sponsors conferences and workshops offering not only the findings from center's research but training in its research methodologies.

From the perspective of a health data user, there are other resources that the Center can offer. By contacting the appropriate NCHS division it is possible to obtain detailed statistics, many unpublished, on the topics for which the Center compiles data. Center staff are also available to help with methodological issues and provide that "one number" that the health data analyst may require. In short, the NCHS is a service-oriented agency that serves a number of invaluable functions for those who require data on health and healthcare. Additional information is available on the NCHS at www.cdc.gov/nchs.

Community Surveys

The other primary source method of case-finding is through the administration of community surveys. The community survey method involves the interviewing and/ or clinical examination of a sample of the population under study. Since many cases are not diagnosed and/or treated, reported cases are likely to represent only a fraction of the total cases of the condition in question. Sample surveys represent an alternative source of data, one that hopefully reveals the "true" prevalence of disease. Surveys provide a mechanism for identifying the totality of morbid conditions within a population, thereby supplementing the knowledge gained by studying reported cases.

Information might be collected from the study population on existing symptoms, conditions previously diagnosed, any treatment received, and any other factor appropriate for determining the extent of morbidity and disability within the population. Clinicians may be involved in the survey process in order to perform examinations or diagnostic procedures. The objective is to identify all cases of the condition under study within the population, not just those that have come to the attention of the various reporting mechanisms.

One approach used in sample surveys is to question respondents with regard to their health status and level of morbidity. The most direct—and the most subjective—approach to measuring health status involves self-assessments by survey respondents. Various community surveys have employed "global" indicators as a means of measuring health status based on self-reports. The major government study to take this approach is the NHIS. With global indicators, survey respondents are typically asked to rate their health status on some type of scale.

While self-reported ratings of health status are attractive in their simplicity, critics contend that they are too subjective. Indeed, the discussion in Chap. 2 of what constitutes health and illness clearly points to the dangers of this approach. One respondent's ill-health may be another's normal state, and it is difficult to control for these variations in perception. Recent research has found, in fact, that African-American respondents and white respondents use a different framework for their self-evaluation, thereby limiting the value of comparative data (Brandon and Proctor 2010). Another review of four different sources of self-reported health status concluded that the results were too inconsistent to be considered accurate indicators of population health (Salomon et al. 2009).

A reasonable correlation has been found, however, between self-reported ratings of health status and more objectively derived indicators of health status. When self-assessments are correlated with responses to a symptom checklist, for example, a relatively strong correlation is evidenced (Proctor et al. 1998). That is, respondents with a large number of symptoms (either self-reported or observed) tend to rate their health status lower than those with few identified symptoms. Self-reported health status has even been shown to be a strong predictor of subsequent mortality (Moesgaard-Iburg et al. 2002). The landmark analysis by Rogers et al. (2000) found a high correlation between self-assessed health status and mortality rates.

The use of symptom checklists in sample surveys is another approach to the development of morbidity indicators. A list of symptoms that has been statistically validated is utilized to collect data for the calculation of a morbidity index. These checklist items are used to derive health status measures for both physical and mental illness (Sacker et al. 2003). There are usually 15 to 20 symptoms, since it is difficult to retain respondents' attention for much longer than that. While the symptoms are sometimes examined individually, the main use is in the calculation of an index. Typically, the number of symptoms is simply summed and this becomes the index score for that individual. In some cases, the symptoms may be weighted on the grounds that some symptoms are more important in the determination of morbidity levels than others.

A primary rationale for the utilization of symptom checklists is the fact that much of the population is free of clinically identifiable disorders but is likely to have some, albeit minor, manifestations of ill-health. Virtually everyone has vaguely defined symptoms of some type at various times or clearly identifiable ones that cannot be linked to a particular clinical condition. It is further argued, with regard to both physical and mental conditions, that these "everyday" symptoms are more significant measures of health status than are the comparatively rare clinical conditions. Symptom checklists are also attractive because of their objective nature and generally agreed-upon definitions. Virtually everyone is going to agree as to what constitutes an "occasional cough" or "occasional dizzy spells," but clinical diagnoses are often misunderstood by patients or obscured by the terminological complexity of the healthcare setting.

Symptom checklists are used to obtain answers directly from survey respondents. Respondents either complete a questionnaire that contains the checklist or provide responses to an interviewer who records them. In some rare cases, the checklist will include signs as well as symptoms, and clinical personnel will be involved in the data collection process to obtain test results ("signs"). This approach is occasionally utilized, for example, in studies of psychiatric morbidity, in which case the clinician will typically administer one or more psychometric tests. The index calculated in this manner generally reflects a combination of symptoms reported by the respondent and signs observed by the clinician. The morbidity profiles of the individuals within a population can be combined to create a cumulative profile for the population. This allows for the development of an overall morbidity rate for that population (often presented in terms of an incidence or prevalence rate). Exhibit 4.3 presents an example of a symptom checklist.

Exhibit 4.3: Sample Symptom Checklist

The following checklist is representative of the types of items that might be included in a physical health assessment:

- Abdominal pain
- Blood in stool

(continued)

Exhibit 4.3 (continued)

- Chest pain
- Constipation
- Cough
- Diarrhea
- Difficulty swallowing
- Dizziness
- Eye discomfort and redness
- Foot pain or ankle pain
- Foot swelling or leg swelling
- Headaches
- Heart palpitations
- Hip pain
- Knee pain
- Low back pain
- Nasal congestion
- Nausea or vomiting
- Neck pain
- Numbness or tingling in hands
- Pelvic pain: female
- Pelvic pain: male
- Shortness of breath
- Shoulder pain
- Sore throat
- Urinary problems
- Vision problems
- Wheezing

Source: Mayo Clinic

Respondents may also be asked about their morbidity history. This would include questions about previous diagnoses of various diseases (e.g., diabetes, heart disease, asthma, or some other condition), if they are currently being treated for a certain condition, or if a physician had ever told them they were obese or affected by some other condition. These are typical questions from the Behavioral Risk Factor Surveillance System (BRFSS) interview form fielded by the CDC. For many purposes, the BRFSS is the most useful survey for identifying the health status of various populations.

The National Health Interview Survey (NHIS) in which data are collected annually from approximately 50000 households, is perhaps the center's most important survey. The NHIS is the nation's primary source of data on the incidence/prevalence of health conditions, health status, the injuries and disabilities characterizing the population, health services utilization, and a variety of other health-related topics. Because of the limitations of survey administration, however, the NHIS can only collect data on a relatively handful of the thousands of potential diagnoses.

Unfortunately, the data available on psychiatric morbidity is much less plentiful than that on physical health conditions. What little epidemiologists know about the level and nature of mental disorders within the population has been derived from community surveys. Much useful information on the distribution of mental disorders within US society was generated by the federally funded Epidemiological Catchment Area Study conducted from 1980 to 1985 (Regier et al. 1984). Data were collected from a sample of residents in five-sites across the nation using the Diagnostic Interview Schedule (DIS). The DIS was based on clinical criteria described in the Diagnostic and Statistical Manual (version III) and has generally been abandoned in favor of other screening instruments.

The only current efforts toward systematic nationwide identification and measurement of psychiatric morbidity are the NHIS and the CDC's BRFSS. The former includes considerably more detail in terms of inquiries related to morbidity status. Although both surveys are administered annually, the survey items may vary from year to year. In the case of the BRFSS survey, some of the survey items are optional and participating entities (e.g., states) may or may not opt for certain items. Current survey items on the NHIS-fielded survey related to past diagnosis of mental conditions, recent experiences with cognitive impairment and substance use/abuse, and feelings of emotional discomfort, among others. Current (2012) NHIS survey items related to mental health are presented in Exhibit 4.4.

Exhibit 4.4: Mental Health-Related Items. National Health Interview Survey 2012

The 2012 NHIS interview schedule included the following mental health-related items (in some cases paraphrased for greater readability):
Have you ever been told by a doctor or other health professional that you had...

- Phobia or fears?
- Attention deficit hyperactivity disorder (ADHD) or attention deficit disorder (ADD)?
- Bipolar disorder?
- Depression?
- Other mental health disorders?

During (specified time period), have you experienced...

- Memory loss or loss of other cognitive functions?
- Neurological problems?
- Excessive use of alcohol or tobacco?
- Substance abuse, other than alcohol or tobacco?

During (specified time period), have you felt...

- Anxious, nervous, or worried?
- Stressed?

(continued)

Exhibit 4.4   (continued)

- So sad that nothing could cheer you up?
- Nervous?
- Restless or fidgety?
- Hopeless?
- That everything was an effort?
- Worthless?

How much did these feelings interfere with your life or activities?
How long have you had a developmental problem (e.g., cerebral palsy)?
How long have you had intellectual disability, also known as mental retardation?
How long have you had senility?
How long have you had depression, anxiety, or an emotional problem?
Did you fail to obtain mental healthcare or counseling because you couldn't afford it?
During (specified time period), have you seen or talked to a mental health professional such as a psychiatrist, psychologist, psychiatric nurse, or clinical social worker?

The behavioral health issues addressed by the BRFSS include questions with regard to the number of days (within a specified period) of good mental health, the number of days that physical or mental health problems kept the respondents from doing their usual activities, such as self-care, work, or recreation, the presence of frequent mental distress or serious psychological distress, and whether or not mental health treatment had been received. Exhibit 4.5 presents mental health-related items available through the BRFSS.

Exhibit 4.5: Mental Health-Related Questions. Behavioral Risk Factor Surveillance System

The following questions are available for inclusion in BRFSS surveys (in some cases paraphrased for greater readability):

Now thinking about your mental health, which includes stress, depression, and problems with emotions, for how many days during the past 30 days was your mental health not good?
During (specified time period), for about how many days did poor physical or mental health keep you from doing your usual activities, such as self-care, work, or recreation?
During (specified time period), have you experienced frequent mental distress?

(continued)

Exhibit 4.5 (continued)

During (specified time period), have you experienced serious psychological distress?
During (specified time period), have you received mental health treatment or medicine?
About how often (all of the time, most of the time, some of the time, a little of the time, or none of the time) during (specified time period) did you feel ...

- Nervous?
- Hopeless?
- Restless or fidgety?
- So depressed that nothing could cheer you up?
- That everything was an effort?
- Worthless?

During (specified time period), for about how many days did a mental health condition or emotional problem keep you from doing your work or other usual activities?
Are you now taking medicine or receiving treatment from a doctor or other health professional for any type of mental health condition or emotional problem?
To what extent do you agree that treatment can help people with mental illness lead normal lives?
To what extent do you agree that people are generally caring and sympathetic to people with mental illness?

As noted previously, disability as a measure of morbidity is particularly difficult to operationalize since what is considered a handicap can be highly subjective. The extent of this definitional problem has been recognized by the US Census Bureau, which (after an unsuccessful data collection attempt in 1970) decided to discontinue its question on disability. Another attempt at calculating the level of functional disability and activity limitations within the population was made with the 1990 census. As a result of the challenges in defining disability in terms of specific handicaps, students of disability long ago ceased thinking of disability in terms of specific physical or mental conditions. Most researchers have reconceptualized disability in terms of the consequences of a condition. In the NHIS, "limitation of activity" refers to a long-term reduction in a person's capacity to perform the usual kind or amount of activities associated with his or her age group due to a chronic condition.

This definitional problem is partly resolved by the utilization of more objective and easily measured indicators as proxies for disability (as discussed in Chap. 2). One category of indicators focuses on "activities of daily living" (ADL). ADLs constitute a series of indicators related to the ability of individuals to care for themselves, solely or with assistance. Thus, the respondent is asked to what extent he can feed himself, dress himself, and go to the bathroom unassisted. Other indicators may address mobility, as in the ability to climb stairs, walk a certain distance without discomfort, and so forth. ADLs offer a fairly effective means of getting at the overall disability status of individuals by combining their responses into a score that indicates the individual's relative level of disability.

The primary ongoing source of data on disability is the American Community Survey (ACS) (Siordia and Young 2013). The ACS adopted the disability questions being developed for the Census 2000 sample survey. Those questions were modified slightly in 2003 to address an issue with the skip pattern, but otherwise attempted to capture the same population. The types of disability captured through this survey included: sensory disability (e.g., blindness, hearing impairment), physical disability (e.g., limitations in walking, lifting), mental disability (e.g., emotional condition, learning difficulties), self-care disability (e.g., problems with dressing, bathing), go-outside-the-home disability (e.g., activity restrictions due to a disability), and employment disability (e.g., limitations on the ability to work).

The ACS went into full production in 2005, sampling 250000 households per month and producing estimates for geographies with populations of 65000 or greater. The disability items focused on the presence of specific conditions, rather than the impact those conditions might have on basic functioning. An interagency group was formed to develop a new set of questions. In 2006, the Census Bureau fielded a Content Test to assess new and modified content for the ACS questionnaire. The modified disability questions were tested against the existing set of questions and new questions introduced in 2008. Because of the changes to the questions, the new ACS disability questions should not be compared to the previous ACS disability questions or the Census 2000 disability data.

The questionnaire items introduced in 2008 are included in the current ACS questionnaires. They cover the following six disability types:

- *Hearing difficulty.* Deaf or having serious difficulty hearing (DEAR).
- *Vision difficulty.* Blind or having serious difficulty seeing, even when wearing glasses (DEYE).
- *Cognitive difficulty.* Because of a physical, mental, or emotional problem, having difficulty remembering, concentrating, or making decisions (DREM).
- *Ambulatory difficulty.* Having serious difficulty walking or climbing stairs (DPHY).
- *Self-care difficulty.* Having difficulty bathing or dressing (DDRS).
- *Independent living difficulty.* Because of a physical, mental, or emotional problem, having difficulty doing errands alone such as visiting a doctor's office or shopping (DOUT).

Respondents who report any one of the six disability types are considered to have a disability.

The NCHS also collects data on disability through the NHIS. The 2012 interview form included a number of items meant to determine the level of disability characterizing community residents as opposed to those who were formally diagnosed and/or treated (National Center for Health Statistics 2013). Exhibit 4.6 presents the NHIS survey items used to measure adult disability.

Exhibit 4.6: NHIS Disability Items

The following items related to adult disability were included in the 2012 NHIS instrument:

- Are you deaf or do you have serious difficulty hearing?
- Are you blind or do you have serious difficulty seeing even when wearing glasses?
- Because of a physical, mental, or emotional condition, do you have serious difficulty concentrating, remembering, or making decisions?
- Do you have serious difficulty walking or climbing stairs?
- Do you have difficulty dressing or bathing?
- Because of a physical, mental, or emotional condition, do you have difficulty doing errands alone such as visiting a doctor's office or shopping?

Source: National Center for Health Statistics

Ultimately, the process of case-finding in order to determine morbidity patterns for a population is a complex one and faces many challenges. Whether identifying morbid individuals and summing this information up to some aggregate level or deriving rates from repositories of known cases, a number of issues must be considered. The reported cases method of identifying cases holds much promise in that every official case must be recorded somewhere to make it qualify as a case. However, reported cases are just that—only cases that have been reported to healthcare entities. Many individuals with clinically identifiable conditions are never diagnosed and, thus, never become part of the morbidity record. For those that are reported, there is no mechanism for compiling from disparate sources data. Instead, it is necessary to rely on the surveys conducted by the NCHS to develop estimates of the level of morbidity characterizing the population.

The community survey method represents an attempt to overcome the deficiencies of the reported cases method and to generate an estimate of "true" prevalence. The NHIS and the Behavioral Risk Surveillance System are the primary examples of community surveys. This method provides a different perspective from the reported cases method, although it is not possible through community surveys to generate the level of detail that can be produced through analysis of reported cases. Nevertheless, much of what we know about population health—particularly with regard to psychiatric morbidity—has been derived from community surveys.

Neither method is sufficient to provide the total picture when it comes to morbidity. It is necessary to use both methods in order to develop a more complete understanding of current morbidity patterns. With improved computer technology and federally sponsored efforts toward the creation of repositories of patient data, an opportunity exists to advance efforts to determine morbidity patterns for the population.

References

Berger, J. T. (2008). The influence of physicians' demographic characteristics and their patients' demographic characteristics on physician practice: Implications for education and research. *Academic Medicine, 83*(1), 100–105.

Brandon, L. J., & Proctor, L. (2010). Comparison of health perceptions and health status in African-Americans and Caucasians. *Journal of the National Medical Association, 102*(7), 590–597.

Centers for Disease Control and Prevention. (2013). *National notifiable disease surveillance system.* Retrieved from http://wwwn.cdc.gov/nndss/.

Kistler, C. E., Walter, L. C., Mitchell, C. M., & Sloane, P. D. (2010). Patient perceptions of mistakes in ambulatory care. *Archives of Internal Medicine, 170*(16), 1480–1487.

Kituse, J. I., & Cicourel, A. V. (1963). A note on the use of official statistics. *Social Problems, 11*(2), 131–139.

Moesgaard-Iburg, K., Salomon, J. A., Tandon, A., & Murray, C. J. L. (2002). Cross-population comparability of physician-assessed and self-reported measures of health. In C. J. L. Murray, J. A. Salomon, C. D. Mathers, & A. D. Lopez (Eds.), *Summary measures of population health: Concepts, ethics, measurement and applications*. Geneva, Switzerland: World Health Organization.

National Center for Health Statistics. (2013). *2012 National Health Interview Survey (NHIS)*. Retrieved from http://wwwn.cdc.gov/nhis/.

Proctor, S. P., Heeren, T., White, R. F., Wolfe, J., Borgos, M. S., David, J. D., et al. (1998). Health status of Persian Gulf War veterans: Self-reported symptoms, environmental exposure and the effect of stress. *International Journal of Epidemiology, 27*(December), 1000–1010.

Regier, D. A., Myers, J. K., Kramer, M., Robins, L. N., Blazer, D. G., Hough, R. L., et al. (1984). The NIMH epidemiologic catchment area program: Historical context, major objectives, and study population characteristics. *Archives of General Psychiatry, 41*(10), 934–941.

Rogers, R. G., Hummer, R. A., & Nam, C. B. (2000). *Living and dying in the USA: Behavioral, health and social differentials of adult mortality*. New York: Academic.

Sacker, A., Wiggins, R. D., Clark, P., & Bartley, M. (2003). Making sense of symptom checklists: A latent class approach to the first 9 years of the British Household Panel Survey. *Journal of Public Health Medicine, 25*(3), 215–222.

Salomon, J. A., Nordhagen, S., Oza, S., & Murray, C. J. L. (2009). Are Americans feeling less healthy? The puzzle of trends in self-rated health. *American Journal of Epidemiology, 170*(3), 343–351.

Senathirajah, M., Owens, P., Mutter, R., & Nagamine, M. (2011). *Special study on the meaning of the first-listed diagnosis on emergency department and ambulatory surgery records* (HCUP Methods Series Report #2011-03).

Siordia, C., & Young, R. (2013). Methodological note: Allocation of disability items in the American Community Survey. *Disability and Health Journal, 6*(2), 149–153.

Additional Resources

Behavioral Risk Factor Surveillance System (BRFSS). Retrieved from http://www.cdc.gov/brfss/

Centers for Disease Control and Prevention. (2013). *Morbidity and Mortality Weekly Report (MMWR)*. Retrieved from http://www.cdc.gov/mmwr/.

Friis, R. H. (2009). *Epidemiology 101*. Burlington, MA: Jones and Bartlett.

National Center for Health Statistics. Retrieved from www.cdc.gov/nchs.

Chapter 5
Measuring Morbidity

Counting Health Conditions

The most direct measure of morbidity involves the simple counting of cases of recognizable conditions for a specified population or unit of geography. While this approach is straightforward, it raises the question of what to count toward the morbidity level and where to get accurate data. In an ideal world, it would be possible to count all existing cases of morbidity for the target population and generate a meaningful rate. It should be obvious by now that this is not a straightforward proposition. Options with regard to "what" to count include: specific indicators for a particular disease, groupings of indicators for a particular disease, narrow categories of diseases, broad categories of diseases or, finally, global indicators that consider *all* indicators of morbidity.

These options can be illustrated using diabetes as an example. A specific indicator would be the number of cases of adult-onset diabetes without complications. The grouping of indicators related to this would involve a count of adult-onset diabetes with and *without* complications along with juvenile-onset diabetes. A broader

---

This chapter addresses the means used to quantify the level of morbidity within a population once cases have been identified. The various techniques used to measure morbidity are described and the usefulness of various measures considered.

© Springer New York 2016
R.K. Thomas, *In Sickness and In Health*, Applied Demography Series 6,
DOI 10.1007/978-1-4939-3423-2_5

grouping would include metabolic diseases (including diabetes) and an even broader grouping would count all cases of chronic disease (including diabetes). Finally, a global measure would include all indicators of morbidity (including diabetes).

The degree of granularity with regard to the amount of morbidity is a function of the objectives of the analysis. As indicated by the formats of the various classification systems discussed in Chap. 3, diseases of a particular type can be reported separately or grouped with other variations of that same condition. Diabetes affecting those under 17 (Type I) and diabetes affecting persons 17 and over (Type II) could be reported separately or jointly, depending on the objective. Or, for some purposes, one might be interested in reporting out those 17 and over exhibiting diabetes with complications separately from those exhibiting diabetes without complications. (Exhibit 5.1 provides examples of specific diseases and the proportion of the population affected.)

Exhibit 5.1: Estimated Cases of Selected Diseases Among Adults

United States: 2011

Disease	Number of cases[a]	Percent of population[b]
Diabetes	20589	8.6
Ulcers	15502	6.5
Kidney disease	4381	1.9
Liver disease	3016	1.2
Arthritis	53782	22.1
Chronic joint symptoms	68749	28.7

[a]In thousands
[b]Age adjusted
Source: National Center for Health Statistics (2012). Summary of Health Statistics for U.S. Adults: National Health Interview Survey, 2011, *Vital and Health Statistics* Series 10, Number 256

In some cases an analyst may use a specific clinical reading as the indicator of a disease. A good example of this is the use of the body mass index as a measure of obesity. The BMI has come into use as a meaningful single figure for assessing the health status of an individual and, then, aggregating individuals into an obesity rate for the population under study. The BMI is popular because of the ease with which it can be calculated and with which it can be understood. Exhibit 5.2 describes the use of the BMI as a measure of morbidity.

Exhibit 5.2: BMI as a Measure of Morbidity

The steady increase in the collection of healthcare data via disease reports, administrative data, and surveys has made it possible to create a variety of morbidity and comorbidity indices. These indices are subsequently used in a host of analyses designed to provide insights into the changes in the levels of sickness and illness. In addition, the indices are linked to mortality data in order to better understand shifts in death rates (Chaudhry et al. 2005).

One index receiving significant attention in recent years is a simple one, the body mass index (BMI). The BMI is generated through a simple calculation:

$$BMI = \frac{Mass\,(Kg\,or\,pounds)}{(Height\,(m\,or\,inches))^2}$$

The BMI is not a direct measure of morbidity but an indicator of risk for morbid conditions such as high blood pressure and diabetes. BMI scores are classified into seven categories ranging from severely underweight, index score less than 16.5 (e.g., a person who is 5′5″ and weighs less than 118 lb) to Obese Class 3 (e.g., a 5′5″ person weighing 290 pounds or more). BMI scores can be calculated by age, thus allowing for the objective identification of persons who are overweight for their age.

It should be noted that the BMI has several shortcomings. The BMI sometimes overestimates adiposity in those who have more lean body mass and underestimates adiposity in those who have less lean body mass. For example, those with intermediate BMI scores are sometimes found to have high risk of death from diseases such as coronary artery disease than those with higher BMI scores (Romero-Corral et al. 2008). These shortcomings limit its usefulness for predictive modeling.

The BMI is relatively easy to calculate and comparing scores over time provides a good summary of the growing problem of obesity in the United States and other developed countries. By examining shifts over time in the distribution of BMI scores among children in the United States, health researchers have been able to document the growing epidemic of childhood obesity. The importance of obesity as a precursor to a variety of health conditions makes this simple index invaluable.

References

Chaudhry, Saima, Jin, Lei and Meltzer, David (2005). Use of a self-report-generated Charlson comorbidity index for predicting mortality. *Medical Care* 43(6): 607–615.

Romero-Corral, A., Somers, V. K., Sierra-Johnson, J., Thomas, R. J., Collazo-Clavell, M. L., Korinek, J., Allison, T. G., and Batsis, J. A. (2008). Accuracy of body mass index in diagnosing obesity in the adult general population. *International Journal of Obesity* 32(6): 959–956.

In some cases a category of diseases may be identified as a measure of morbidity rather than specific diseases. For example, one may determine the overall incidence of acute conditions or the overall prevalence of chronic conditions. This approach might be taken when less specificity is required or when these categories provide a useful depiction of the population's health status. Other examples of categories of disease that might be considered are reproductive health problems, childhood diseases, or mental health disorders.

As noted previously, more than one diagnosis may be assigned to a patient or case. A primary diagnosis is typically attached to the individual based on presenting symptoms. This primary diagnosis is referred to as the "first-listed" diagnosis in a medical record. In calculating the amount of morbidity characterizing a population, analysts may consider either the first-listed diagnoses or any-listed diagnosis, depending on their objectives (Senathirajah et al. 2011). Obviously, counting all diagnoses will yield a much larger number of conditions (and certainly more conditions than there are patients) and a truer picture of the morbidity of the population than would using only the first-listed diagnosis. The decision to use only one diagnosis (the first-listed) or all diagnoses will hinge on the objectives of the analysis. It should be noted, however, morbidity indices for some high acuity conditions may be less reliable and valid due to the presence of complications and comorbidities (Roos et al. 1997).

Calculating Percentages and Rates

While counting morbid cases represents a necessary first step in morbidity analysis, these counts must be converted into some metric that allows comparison. Counts themselves do not mean much unless they can be seen in context. If the goal is to compare two populations or track one population over time, counts have limited usefulness. Conceptually, the morbidity rate is defined as the proportion of the population affected by a disease or diseases and thus measures the frequency with which a disease occurs within that population. This proportion could be expressed as a percentage or a rate. Developing a proportional measure allows for comparisons over time and between populations of different sizes, thereby improving on morbidity assessments based on counts. The number of cases, for example, for communities of very different sizes does not serve well as a comparative measure, whereas a percentage or a rate allows a one-to-one comparison (adjusting, of course, of differences in population composition).

A percentage is perhaps the most intuitive measure in that everyone including laymen understand what this means. As illustrated below, the proportion of the population affected by a health condition can be calculated simply by dividing the number of known cases by the population. Thus, 100 affected people within a population of 1000 generate a morbidity rate of 10 %. To even the casual observer this suggests that one in ten people within this population is affected.

A rate represents a different proportional measure, although reflecting the same concept. A rate could be expressed per 100 people, 1000 people, 10000 people or 100000 people, depending on the morbidity indicator being used. Thus, a global morbidity rate that counted all chronic diseases within a population might be expressed as a number per 100 residents, since the total chronic disease burden is likely to affect a large proportion of the population. On the other hand, a relatively rare disease (e.g., sickle cell anemia) might more reasonably be expressed as a rate per 100000.

In actual practice, there are a variety of morbidity rates to choose from. The calculation of morbidity rates requires information on the number of identified cases for the disease(s) in question (the numerator) and the number of people at risk for contracting that disease or diseases (the denominator). The numerator—that is, the existing number of cases of the condition within the denominator—would be drawn from epidemiological data (with all the caveats that implies). The denominator in this equation—the population at risk—is usually readily available since it is typically a known quantity. The population at risk is the number of persons who have some nonzero probability of contracting the condition in question. As noted elsewhere, identifying the population at risk is often a challenge in its own right.

Rates may be calculated using a variety of different figures for the denominator (i.e., the population at risk). For many conditions, the population at risk is synonymous with the total population, and the infection rate is relatively easy to calculate. For a condition that is pandemic—e.g., seasonal flu—essentially the entire population is at risk. Thus, the CDC calculates the influenza rate using the number of new cases identified for a specified time period and assumes that the total population is at risk.

This approach, however, may generate a rate that would be considered too "crude" to support a meaningful interpretation. It is seldom the case, in fact, that the total population is at risk. Selective risk has become more common as chronic diseases—particularly those that are lifestyle related—have come to dominate the morbidity spectrum. Certain subsets of the population may have a predisposition toward a specific disease (e.g., African-Americans and sickle cell anemia), be at risk due to selective exposure (e.g., coal miners and black lung disease), attend the same event (e.g., food poisoning at a banquet), or practice risky behavior (e.g., male homosexuals and HIV/AIDS). For these reasons the specification of the denominator may be a challenge, requiring the analyst to have an in-depth understanding of the health condition under study.

The examples below present morbidity calculations with the results shown as a percent:

$$\text{Morbidity rate} = \frac{\text{Number of cases of disease}_x \text{ during time}_x}{\text{Population at risk during time}_x} = \underline{\quad} \%$$

$$\text{Morbidity rate} = \frac{100 \text{ Cases of asthma}}{1000} = 10.0 \%$$

The examples below present morbidity calculations with the results shown as a rate:

$$\text{Morbidity rate} = \frac{\text{Number of cases of disease}_x \text{ during time}_x}{\text{Population at risk at time}_x} \times 1000 = \underline{\quad\quad} / 1000$$

$$\text{Morbidity rate} = \frac{100 \text{ Cases of asthma}}{1000} = \times 1000 = 100/1000$$

It may be that the overall morbidity rate is not precise enough. Two measures used by epidemiologists for quantifying the level of morbidity—incidence and prevalence rates—represent variations on the morbidity rate. An *incidence rate* refers to the number of new cases of a disease or condition identified over a certain time period expressed as a proportion of the population at risk. Incidence rates are calculated by dividing the number of reported cases during a specific time period by the population at risk. A *prevalence rate* represents the totality of morbidity at a specific point in time. The prevalence rate is calculated by dividing the total number of persons with the disease or condition in question by the population at risk at a specific point in time. Thus, the prevalence rate includes all cases extant at a point in time (i.e., existing cases plus newly diagnosed cases). The prevalence rate typically exceeds the incidence rate, since the latter is but a fraction of the former. The only time the two rates are nearly comparable is when the condition is acute and of very short duration. For example, the incidence rate would almost equal the prevalence rate at the height of a 24-hour virus epidemic since victims recover almost as quickly as they are affected.

The calculation of the incidence and prevalence rates for AIDS illustrates the use of the two different rates. The incidence rate for persons diagnosed as having AIDS in 2005 in the United States was:

$$\frac{\text{AIDS cases diagnosed during 2005}}{\text{Population at risk mid} - 2005} = \text{Cases per 100000 population}$$

The prevalence rate for AIDS at the end of 2005, on the other hand, would be calculated as follows:

$$\frac{\text{AIDS cases diagnosed during 2005} + \text{existing cases of AIDS}}{\text{Population at risk at the end of 2005}} = \text{Cases per 100000}$$

$$\text{population}$$

The incidence rate is a valuable measure in epidemiological investigations. If a new or mysterious condition afflicts a population, epidemiologists can trace the spread of the condition through the population by backtracking using incidence data. The cause or population of origin of a new disease can often only be determined by identifying the characteristics of the victims and the conditions under which the disease was contracted. The exact date of occurrence becomes crucial if the epidemiological detective is to link the onset of the disease to a particular set of circumstances. AIDS is a case in point wherein the means of transmission may be identified based on the characteristics of the affected individuals.

The prevalence rate can be used in much the same way when the condition is a chronic one. There is less interest in determining the origin and progression of a disorder within a population than in determining the number of patients with that condition within a population at a given point in time. This is precisely how many hospitals and other healthcare providers forecast demand for their services.

Incidence and prevalence rates can both be used to generate estimates and projections of the level of morbidity. If the analyst knows, for example, that the incidence rate for a certain condition is 17 per 1000 population aged 65 years and over and has reason to believe that the incidence rate for that condition will remain nearly constant for the next 5 years (data must support this assumption), then the number of cases 5 years in the future can be determined by multiplying the incidence rate by the projected population of persons age 65 and above. The prevalence rate can be used in much the same way when the condition is a chronic one. A formula like the following might be used to estimate the number of cases expected for a particular condition (in this example a chronic disease):

$$\text{Expected case} = (\frac{\text{Rate} / 1000 \times \text{population}}{1000})$$

$$\text{Expected case of diabetes} = (\frac{\text{Diabetes rate} / 1000 \times \text{population}}{1000})$$

or

$$\text{Expected cases of diabetes} = (\frac{150 / 1000 \times 10000}{1000}) = 1500 \text{ cases}$$

This example represents a relatively "crude" view of a morbidity rate since it does not take into account the demographic makeup of the population in question. For many health conditions a rate calculated based on the total population may not be appropriate. If data are available a better estimate can be generated by using rates specific to age, sex, race, or some other factor known to affect the amount of morbidity attributable to the condition under study. At a minimum, it would be desirable to adjust the estimates for the age structure and sex breakdown for the population being analyzed. A simple example is presented below in which broad age groups and sex are factored into the estimate.

Age group	Males	Male rate	Cases	Females	Female rate	Cases	Total cases
0–14	525	0.0	0	475	20.0	10	10
15–24	500	30.0	15	500	35.0	18	33
25–44	1400	60.0	84	1500	70.0	105	189
45–64	1800	200.0	360	2300	275.0	632	992
65 and over	400	350.0	140	600	450.0	270	410
Total	4625		599	5375		1035	1634

In this example, the calculations yield an overall rate of 163.4 per 1000 and a total of 1634 cases, a figure somewhat higher than the global rate if the prevalence rate for the total population were to be used. The refined estimate reflects an older, predominantly female population exhibiting a higher than average rate. (Rates of diabetes prevalence by age and sex were drawn from the National Ambulatory Medical Care Survey conducted annually by the National Center for Health Statistics.)

A related measure that might be utilized is the *proportional morbidity rate* or the proportion of *all* diseased individuals in the population with the particular disease under discussion. In this case, the denominator is not the total population but the population of affected individuals. Among the population with any chronic disease, for example, what proportion suffers from diabetes? The proportional morbidity rate is calculated using the following formula:

$$\text{Proportional morbidity ratio} = \frac{\text{Number of cases of a specified condition during time}_x}{\text{Total cases during time}_x}$$

Using a concrete example, the following proportional morbidity rate is generated:

$$\text{Proportional morbidity ratio} = \frac{100 \text{ Diabetes cases during time period x}}{1000 \text{ Total cases during time period x}} = 10.0$$

The proportional morbidity ratio can be used to compare the relative morbidity for two populations by simply dividing the PMR for Population A by the PMR for Population B. This generates a proportional morbidity ratio. To wit:

$$\text{Comparative morbidity ratio} = \frac{\text{PMR}_{\text{PopA}}}{\text{PMR}_{\text{PopB}}} = \underline{\qquad}$$

or

$$\text{Comparative morbidity ratio} = \frac{10}{15} = 0.67$$

The PMR can also be used to track changes in morbidity levels over time by comparing the PMR for a population for two or more time periods.

This measure could also be considered an indicator of *relative risk* or the ratio of two incidence or prevalence rates. Typically, the rate for the population being analyzed would be divided by the rate for a control or reference population. Relative risk is useful for comparing populations affected by a certain condition to populations not affected by that condition. For example, the prevalence rate for asthma in a city characterized by a high level of air pollution might be compared to the rate for a city with a low level of pollution. Dividing the rate for the former by the rate for the latter will generate a measure of relative risk.

One other way of looking at the likelihood of one population being affected compared to other populations is through the calculation of *odds ratios*. The odds represent the chances of one population having a condition compared to the chances in other populations—e.g., the chances of being exposed to a disease in one population compared to the chances of exposure in another population. As with relative risk, the calculation involves dividing the odds for one population by the odds for another population. For calculating relative risk and odds ratios, the numerators are the same; it is the denominators that differ.

It is sometimes necessary to standardize the morbidity rate so that it is expressed as a proportion of the expected rate compared with a standard group. Standardization is necessary when two or more populations are being compared in terms of their morbidity status or when a population's morbidity status is being analyzed over time. A general morbidity rate, while useful for some purposes, may offer a misleading view of a population's morbidity status if the population does not exhibit a "normal" demographic profile.

A case in point involves the state of Florida where morbidity rates for chronic disease are found to be inordinately high. These rates defy the conventional wisdom that Florida is a healthy place to live. Even a casual observer is likely to note the "abnormal" age structure of the state's population, since Florida exhibits a much older age structure than the nation as a whole. In order to determine the "true" overall morbidity rate or the rates for specific diseases, the population structure must be statistically adjusted to resemble some "standard" population (most often the US population). Once the age structure has been standardized, new morbidity rates can be calculated that represent a more accurate depiction of the state's actual morbidity level.

This approach is referred to as *direct standardization. Indirect standardization* involves a similar methodology but, in that case, the morbidity rate for each disease (rather than the population) is adjusted to reflect a more "normal" disease rate. This produces the number of "expected cases" that can then be compared to the number of "observed cases," allowing the analyst to draw conclusions about the morbidity status of the two populations based on the differences between expected cases and observed cases. Exhibit 5.3 describes the process used to standardize health data.

Exhibit 5.3: Standardization of Health Data

Standardization is a method used by epidemiologists and population scientists to adjust measures of vital processes for compositional factors that have an effect on those rates. The number of cases of disease occurring in any year is a function of three components: health status, population size, and demographic attributes (e.g., age). In comparing morbidity rates for two or more populations, it is important to hold population size and age structure (and perhaps other attributes) constant when morbidity rates are being constructed.

The calculation of rates addresses concerns over differences in population size and allows the analyst to compare the health status of two populations that are different demographically. A basic morbidity rate that uses the total population as the denominator is likely to be the first rate calculated. However, the overall morbidity rate may be misleading since the level of morbidity is influenced by differences in the age structures of the populations in question. That is, areas

(continued)

Exhibit 5.3 (continued)

with relatively young populations (and hence less risk of chronic disease) are likely to report low morbidity rates, while areas with relatively old populations (and greater risk of chronic disease) are likely to report high morbidity rates independent of the size of the respective populations. For this reason, the unadjusted morbidity rate is not a good measure for comparative purposes.

It is possible to adjust or standardize rates in order to control for age structure and, often, other factors (e.g., race). One method for accomplishing this is to select a "standard" age structure (e.g., the age structure for the United States), apply the incidence rate from two different populations to the standard age distribution, and then compare the number of cases after the adjustment. This process generates the number of cases for the respective populations *as if* their age structures were the same. The revised number of deaths (the numerator) can then be divided by the population and an age-adjusted morbidity rate generated.

Standardizing the incidence rate for diabetes

Age group	Community population	Rate[a]	Cases	Standard population	Rate[a]	Cases
0–14	13000	15.0	195	5000	15.0	75
15–24	12000	30.0	360	5000	30.0	150
25–44	10000	65.0	650	14500	65.0	9425
45–64	8000	250.0	2000	15500	250.0	3875
65 and over	7000	425.0	2975	5000	425.0	2125
Total	50000		6180			15650
Prevalence rate:	123.6/1000			313.0/1000		

[a]Rate per 1000 population

Using a specific disease as an example, the following table illustrates a method for adjusting the incidence rate for a particular population.

An inspection of the data indicates that the community exhibits a very young population reporting relatively few cases of diabetes. However, when this community's population is adjusted to resemble a more "normal" population, the number of expected cases increases dramatically, and the prevalence rate increases from 123.6 to 313.0 per 1000.

Demographers distinguish between "direct" and "indirect" standardization to refer to the use of two different ways in which to account for differences in age structure. Direct standardization is used to calculate a weighted average of the age-specific rates of the population under study where the weights represent the age-specific sizes of the *standard* population. Indirect standardization is used to produce age-specific rates from the *standard* population to derive expected cases in the population under study. In this method, the morbidity rate of the population is multiplied by an adjustment factor that is designed to take account of the peculiarities of the age composition or age-sex composition, of the population of the community.

(continued)

Exhibit 5.3 (continued)

The same principles of standardization can be used to adjust rates for other factors, such as education, race, and ethnicity. A similar process can be utilized to adjust mortality rates by holding certain factors constant. For example, the death rates for a predominantly white population and a predominantly African-American population might be recalculated using a standardized method that assumes that the populations have comparable racial characteristics.

Two additional rates utilized by demographers are case rates and case fatality rates. A *case rate* is merely an expression of the reported incidence of a disease per 1000, 10000, or 100000 persons and is not as finely tuned as a rate that is adjusted for the population at risk. This is comparable to the basic morbidity rate described above. The *case fatality rate* is generated by dividing the number of persons who die from a certain disease by the number of persons who contracted that disease. The quotient is expressed as a percentage. For example, through 1996, 7629 children had contracted AIDS and 4406, about 58 %, had died.

Often, cohorts of persons first diagnosed with a disease are followed through time—and in some cases to death—in order to track the progression of the disease or the response to various treatment modalities. In one study successive cohorts of pediatric AIDS patients who contracted the disease between 1979 and 1991 were followed over time. Although the case fatality rate was high for all cohorts, median survival time increased over the interval. The increase in survival is linked in part to improvements in pediatric AIDS treatment (Barnhart et al. 1996). It is possible to refine the above rates to include more narrowly defined populations at risk.

Global Measures of Morbidity

The most comprehensive approach to measuring the level of morbidity is through the assessment of the overall health status of the population. Attempts to develop a single indicator of morbidity in terms of health status have not been very successful, and specific measures continue to be utilized as indicators. More recent efforts toward developing a single indicator incorporating measures of mortality and morbidity that reflect healthy life-years have been more successful (Hyder et al. 1998), but no widely accepted overall indicator has emerged.

Indicators of health status that address the overall health condition for individuals or populations are referred to as "global indicators." The most direct—and the most subjective—approach to measuring health status involves self-assessments by survey respondents. With global indicators, survey respondents are typically asked to rate their health status on some type of scale.

Although some scales may be relatively complex, the most common response categories are "poor," "fair," "good," "very good," and "excellent." Once such ratings have been obtained from a number of respondents, assessments of the health status of a population can be performed. Various community surveys have utilized global indicators as a means of measuring health status based on self-reports. The major government study to take this approach is the National Health Interview Survey (NHIS) conducted by the National Center for Health Statistics.

While self-reported ratings of health status are attractive in their simplicity, some consider them too subjective. Indeed, the discussion in Chap. 2 of what constitutes health and illness clearly points to the dangers of this approach. One respondent's ill-health may be another's normal state, and it is difficult to control for these variations in perception. Recent research has found, in fact, that African-American respondents and white respondents use a different framework for their self-evaluation, thereby limiting the value of comparative data (Brandon and Proctor 2010).

These concerns have been partially addressed in that a reasonable correlation has been found between self-reports and objective measures of health status. When self-assessments are correlated with responses to a symptom checklist, for example, a relatively strong correlation is evidenced (Proctor et al. 1998). That is, respondents with a large number of symptoms (either self-reported or observed) tend to rate their health status lower than those with few identified symptoms. Self-reported health status has even been shown to be a strong predictor of subsequent mortality (Moesgaard-Iburg et al. 2002). Exhibit 5.4 presents self-reported rating of health status for selected demographic groups.

Exhibit 5.4: Self-Assessed Health Status for Adults

By selected biosocial characteristics, United States, 2010

Characteristic	Excellent (%)	Very Good (%)	Good (%)	Fair (%)	Poor (%)
Total	36.0	30.4	23.9	7.4	2.2
Age					
Under 12 years	55.7	27.2	15.2	1.8	0.1
12–17 Years	53.8	26.7	17.3	2.0	0.3
18–44 Years	37.4	33.1	23.2	5.3	1.0
45–64 Years	23.7	31.4	28.9	11.6	4.4
65–74 Years	16.6	29.7	32.5	16.0	5.1
75 Years and over	11.6	24.5	35.5	30.6	7.7
Sex					
Male	36.7	30.4	23.7	7.0	2.2
Female	35.3	30.4	24.2	7.8	2.3
Race/ethnicity					
White	37.6	30.9	22.7	6.8	2.1
Black	27.7	36.8	30.5	11.6	3.3
Asian	36.3	30.8	24.8	6.6	1.6
American Indian	22.7	31.7	27.6	13.6	4.4
Hispanic	30.8	27.7	28.5	10.4	2.7

Source: National Center for Health Statistics (2011). *Summary Health Statistics for the U.S. Population: National Health Interview Survey, 2010*. Bethesda, MD: National Center for Health Statistics

A more objective approach to measuring a population's morbidity involves the development of a health status index. Since data on the true incidence/prevalence of morbid conditions are not available and a variety of factors are thought to contribute to a population's health status, the health status index combines a number of indicators thought to have relevance for or to reflect morbidity. Some of these indicators (e.g., the poverty rate) would be considered "proxy" indicators since they are not measures of disease per se but are factors associated with varying levels of morbidity. Exhibit 5.5 addresses the development of a health status index.

Exhibit 5.5: The Health Status Index

One of the greatest challenges in healthcare over the years has been the development of an acceptable health status index. Beginning with the social indicators movement of the 1960s, there has been periodic interest in the development of an index that could be used to represent the health status of a population or a community in either absolute or relative terms.

A health status index is a single figure that represents the morbidity level for the population or community. It involves an attempt to quantify health status in objective and measurable terms. A health status index is constructed by combining a number of individual health status indicators into a single index. This index can then be utilized to compare the level of need from community to community or for a single community over time. It can be used as a basis for setting priorities and evaluating the worthiness of proposed programs. It can also serve as a basis for allocating resources and as a tool for evaluating the effectiveness of existing programs.

A number of conceptual problems surround the development of health status indices. These problems begin with the question of what indicators to include. Many of the indicators that might be included are fairly obvious. Others, such as certain demographic indicators, might not be. The death rate, for example, would be considered a direct indicator of health status. Others might be referred to as "proxy" measures of health status, in that they are not direct indictors of health conditions but can be assumed to indirectly indicate or influence the level of health status within a population.

The major categories of health status indicators utilized include morbidity indicators, outcome indicators, utilization indicators, resource availability indicators, and functional status indicators. Morbidity measures are obvious indicators of health status, since they reflect the prevalence and/or incidence of various conditions, as well as the level of disability within a population. The primary outcome indicator is the mortality rate. Utilization indicators might include hospital admissions or procedures performed. Resource availability measures would include access to hospitals, physicians and various other facilities and services. Measures of functional state represent a form of

(continued)

Exhibit 5.5 (continued)

morbidity measurement. These include a range of measures such as days of work lost, days of school lost, bed-restricted days, activity-restricted days, and so forth.

Once the indicators are selected for inclusion, the analyst is faced with issues of quantification and measurement. Choices must be made between various available metrics. For example, if income or poverty level is to be included as a proxy indicator, the analyst must choose between measures of poverty (e.g., for families, children, the total population), other measures of income (e.g., median household income, per capita income), or some other measure. Decisions must be made even for more direct measures of morbidity (e.g., disease incidence/prevalence rates).

Once variables have been assigned, the question of how to weight the various component indicators is also raised. In the past, for example, the mortality rate might have been considered a critical indicator of morbidity. Today, however, with fewer deaths being recorded, mortality has become a less important reflection of morbidity patterns. There are no simple means for resolving these issues. Every analyst must address them in the best manner possible and carefully document the process that is used in developing the index.

A number of different methodologies can be utilized for this purpose, and the important factor is to come as close to both scientific rigor and face validity as possible. Assuming that all indicators are to be equally weighted, one approach might be to score each indicator on a scale of 1–5 for each geographic unit. Negative characteristics would be scored closer to 1 and positive characteristics closer to 5. The scores for each indicator could be summed and then divided by the number of indicators to provide an average score for each geographic unit somewhere between 1 and 5. It should be noted that the absolute number generated through the process means little; its value is derived from the ability to compare it with other figures. This index number could be used, for example, to compare one community to another or track the health status of a particular community over time.

Health status indices can be calculated for any level of geography for which data are available. However, the smaller the unit of geography the finer the distinction that can be made. Many health planning agencies conduct analyses down to the census tract level, while others utilize the zip code or county as the unit of analysis. The challenge here is the availability of morbidity data for small areas of geography.

The current methodologies for constructing health status indices are certainly not without their critics. There are numerous conceptual, methodological, and practical issues that must be addressed in the development of a health status index. Nevertheless, the need to better understand the health characteristics of a defined population mandates continued efforts toward the development of a defensible health status index.

Measuring Disability

The level of disability within a population is calculated in the same manner as that for disease. Since disabilities are typically chronic, a prevalence rate is usually generated. The availability of data on disability was described in a previous chapter, and the issue becomes one of which of the various measures of disability to use as the numerator in the calculations. (The total population is typically considered the population at risk.)

Most measures of disability are presented as rates or percentages for the population in question. Thus, we might find statistics on the percent of the population with a specified disability (e.g., 3.4 % of Americans have a hearing disability) or as an aggregate figure for all disabilities (e.g., 12.1 % of Americans report *some* disability). These could just as easily be expressed as rates (Exhibit 5.6 presents some statistics on disability generated by the American Community Survey.)

If activities of daily living (ADLs) are used as the indicator, a scale might be used to generate a score for each individual, with these scores combined to yield a score for the population or group under study. A different approach is used when "restriction" measures are used to quantify disability. Disability is thus measeured in terms of average days missed from work, school, etc., or average days of restricted activity (e.g., days restricted to bed).

There is also a proprietary tool for measuring the level of disability in individuals called the "Health Utilities Index" (HUI). The HUI is described as a "multi-attribute health status classification system" that is used to calculate a health-related quality of life score (Horsman et al. 2003). A questionnaire is used to collect data from individuals with the particular survey instrument tailored to the situation. The collected data is used to classify the individual along a number of different dimensions. The survey instrument elicits information on vision, hearing, speech, ambulation, dexterity, emotion, cognition, and pain. The questionnaires are administered to large study populations as well as to individual patients. Since the system is proprietary, there is limited data available for comparing communities or populations on the index.

When all disabilities are taken into account, at least 40 million Americans are considered to be "disabled" and the figure could be as high as 50 million (Field and Jette 2007). Further, evidence suggests an increase in health conditions among children (e.g., asthma, obesity) that portend future disability. While the increase in the number and proportion of disabled within the US population can be partially attributed to increased numbers of lives saved (e.g., prematurity, trauma cases) and better management of life-threatening conditions (e.g., diabetes, heart disease), a recent study indicated that increases in mental and behavioral disorders and musculoskeletal conditions were major contributors to increasing levels of disability. As a result of these trends, the average number of years living with disability (disability adjusted life-years) has become a more significant statistic than years lost to premature mortality (Murray et al. 2013).

Exhibit 5.6: Disability Prevalence

United States: 2011

Type of disability	Percent of population
Visual disability	2.2
Hearing disability	3.4
Ambulatory disability	6.9
Cognitive disability	4.9
Self-care disability	2.7
Independent living disability	5.6
Any disability	12.1

Source: American Community Survey

References

Barnhart, H. X., Blake Caldwell, M., Thomas, P., et al. (1996). Natural history of human immuno-deficiency virus disease in perinatally infected children: An analysis from the pediatric spectrum of disease project. *Pediatrics, 97*(5), 710–716.

Brandon, L. J., & Proctor, L. (2010). Comparison of health perceptions and health status in African-Americans and Caucasians. *Journal of the National Medical Association, 102*(7), 590–597.

Chaudhry, S., Jin, L., & Meltzer, D. (2005). Use of a self-report-generated Charlson comorbidity index for predicting mortality. *Medical Care, 43*(6), 607–615.

Field, M. J., & Jette, A. M. (Eds.). (2007). *The future of disability in America*. Washington, DC: National Academies Press.

Horsman, J., Furlong, W., Feeny, D., & Torrance', G. (2003). The Health Utilities Index (HUI): Concepts, measurement properties and applications. *Health and Quality of Life Outcomes, 1*, 54. Retrieved from http://www.ncbi.nlm.nih.gov/pmc/articles/PMC293474/.

Hyder, A. A., Rotilant, G., & Morrow, R. H. (1998). Measuring the burden of disease: Healthy life years. *American Journal of Public Health, 88*(2), 196–202.

Moesgaard-Iburg, K., Salomon, J. A., Tandon, A., & Murray, C. J. L. (2002). Cross-population comparability of physician-assessed and self-reported measures of health. In C. J. L. Murray, J. A. Salomon, C. D. Mathers, & A. D. Lopez (Eds.), *Summary measures of population health: Concepts, ethics, measurement and applications*. Geneva, Switzerland: World Health Organization.

Murray, C. J., Atkinson, C., Bhalla, K., Birbeck, G., Burstein, R., Chou, D., et al. (2013). The state of US health, 1990–2010: Burden of diseases, injuries and risk factors. *Journal of the American Medical Association, 310*(6), 591–608. Retrieved from http://jama.jamanetwork.com/article.aspx?articleid=1710486&utm_source.

National Center for Health Statistics. (2011). *Summary health statistics for the U.S. population: National health interview survey, 2010*. Bethesda, MD: National Center for Health Statistics.

National Center for Health Statistics. (2012). *Health, United States: 2011*. Hyattsville, MD: National Center for Health Statistics.

Proctor, S. P., Heeren, T., White, R. F., et al. (1998). Health status of Persian Gulf War veterans: Self-reported symptoms, environmental exposure and the effect of stress. *International Journal of Epidemiology, 27*(6), 1000–1010.

Romero-Corral, A., Somers, V. K., Sierra-Johnson, J., Thomas, R. J., Collazo-Clavell, M. L., Korinek, J., et al. (2008). Accuracy of body mass index in diagnosing obesity in the adult general population. *International Journal of Obesity, 32*(6), 959–956.

Roos, L., Stranc, L., James, R., & Li, J. (1997). Complications, comorbidities and mortality: Improving classification and prediction. *Health Services Research, 32*(2), 229–238.

Senathirajah, M., Owens, P., Mutter, R., Nagamine, M. (2011). *Special study on the meaning of the first-listed diagnosis on emergency department and ambulatory surgery records.* 2011. HCUP Methods Series Report #2011-03. Rockville, MD: U.S. Agency for Healthcare Research and Quality.

Additional Resources

Centers for Disease Control and Prevention. (2013). *Morbidity and mortality weekly report* (MMWR). Atlanta, GA: Centers for Disease Control and Prevention. Retrieved from http://www.cdc.gov/mmwr/.

Friis, R. H. (2009). *Epidemiology 101*. Burlington, MA: Jones & Bartlett.

National Center for Health Statistics. Retrieved from www.cdc.gov/nchs.

Chapter 6
Non-demographic Factors Associated with Morbidity

Having laid a foundation of definitions, case-finding methods, and measurement techniques in previous chapters, this chapter considers the range of factors that influence the level and nature of morbidity characterizing a population. Factors considered include genetics, biological pathogens, environment, lifestyles, and medical services.

Introduction

The morbidity pattern characterizing any population will reflect the influence of a variety of factors. While all populations are exposed to one extent or another to each of the factors that is thought to influence morbidity, the relative importance of morbidity-engendering factors will vary over time and from place to place. While the populations of premodern societies were closer to "nature" and, thus, more directly affected by disease vectors in their environments, contemporary societies are characterized by much more complex etiological patterns. As societies evolved over time, the role of various contributors to morbidity changed. Today a number of factors typically interact to create the morbidity patterns exhibited by modern industrial societies. Further, there are often additional factors within the environment that may "trigger" the onset of a disease that would not have otherwise manifested itself.

One of the underpinnings of the medical model is the doctrine of "specific etiology," and this orientation has driven much of the epidemiological enterprise since the rise of modern medicine. This perspective on disease causation reflects attempts by medical scientists to reduce situations down to their most basic component—in this case, the *one* factor that is causing the disease. As early as the 1950s Dubos

© Springer New York 2016
R.K. Thomas, *In Sickness and In Health*, Applied Demography Series 6,
DOI 10.1007/978-1-4939-3423-2_6

(1959) noted that, while the doctrine of specific etiology has led to important theoretical and practical achievements, it has rarely provided a complete account of the causation of disease. Why, for example, do only some people get sick some of the time and others do not? Questions of this type have made researchers realize that an adequate understanding of illness etiology must take into consideration additional factors that contribute to the onset of disease or share responsibility for its emergence. The days are long gone when public health officials could promote "one bug-one drug-one shot." Too many other factors contribute to today's morbidity patterns. Even when a biological pathogen is involved questions are raised with regard to its source, the circumstances of its emergence, and its interaction with other etiological contributors. The historical emphasis on specific illness-producing agents worked relatively well in dealing with infectious diseases but is too simplistic to explain the onset of complex, chronic illnesses.

Decades of research have led to a better understanding of the correlates of morbidity, and much of the conventional wisdom has been challenged. The shift from a predominance of acute conditions to a predominance of chronic conditions signaled a sea change with regard to disease causation. The major killers a century ago (and throughout human history) could almost invariably be attributed to a single factor. Today's major killers, on the other hand, reflect the interaction of a variety of factors, made possible today by a long life that allows prolonged exposure to carcinogens and the development of degenerative diseases. The contemporary approach to etiology argues for a more complex view of disease causation, one that takes into consideration the interdependence of various factors discussed in the sections that follow.

With our growing understanding of contemporary disease etiology, the need for caution in interpreting the relationships between different variables and morbidity patterns has become increasingly apparent. The interplay of the numerous factors that influence morbidity patterns is obviously complex, and studies that simply explore the direct effects of a particular variable on health status without controlling for the influence of other factors may generate misleading results. Quite often, it has been found that, when additional variables are controlled for, the impact of the original variable is reduced, eliminated, or otherwise modified.

Genetic Factors

Genetic factors are perhaps the most easily identified of the various contributors to morbidity. Among the many determining factors under consideration heredity is, in the case of each individual, the one factor which cannot be intentionally altered. Humans are born with a certain genetic makeup which, while heavily influenced by environmental factors, assigns permanent attributes to each individual. Some of the more significant of these attributes will be clearly evident and play a dominant role in peoples' lives, irrespective of their conditions of existence. A person's appearance—height, hair color, skin color, and eye color—are determined by his or her genes. Mental abilities and natural talents are also affected by heredity, as is the susceptibility to acquire certain diseases.

A genetic disorder is a disease caused in whole or in part by a change in the individual's normal DNA sequence and genome research has indicated that nearly all diseases have a genetic component. Genetic disorders can be caused by a mutation in one gene (monogenic disorder), by mutations in multiple genes (multifactorial inheritance disorder), by a combination of gene mutations and environmental factors, or by damage to chromosomes (National Genome Research Institute 2013). Examples of multifactoral inheritance disorders include many commonly occurring diseases, such as heart disease and diabetes, which are present in many people in different populations around the world.

Genetic disorders such as sickle cell disease, cystic fibrosis, and Tay–Sachs disease typically involve the inheritance of a particular mutated disease-causing gene. The mutated gene is passed down through a family, and each generation of children can inherit the gene that causes the disease. On rare occasions monogenic diseases can occur spontaneously in a child when his/her parents do not carry the affected gene or there is no history of the disease in the family. This can result from a new mutation occurring in the egg or sperm that gave rise to that child. Some disorders develop spontaneously when disease-causing mutations occur during cell division. A modified gene may have no consequence for a person's health or well being, be of minor consequence, or have a dramatic effect on the quality or length of life.

In many disorders genetic and environmental factors work together to bring about changes in otherwise normal genes. For example, some forms of radiation or chemicals may cause cancer in people who are susceptible due to their genetic makeup. Subtle differences in genetic factors will cause people to respond differently to the same environmental exposure. This explains why some individuals have a fairly low risk of developing a disease as a result of an environmental insult, while others are much more vulnerable (National Institute of Environmental Health Sciences 2013).

It is well known that members of certain racial groups are more immune or more susceptible to certain diseases than other races. Further, some diseases, gout and hemophilia, for example, occur regularly in certain families. At one time the belief in heredity was carried so far that it was thought that a disease such as tuberculosis was entirely hereditary. We now know, of course, that none of the infectious diseases are hereditary but are due to contact with a pathogen. Exhibit 6.1 presents examples of diseases attributed to genetic factors.

Exhibit 6.1 Genetic Disease Categorization

Genetics plays a role in thousands of diseases, and a number of factors determine the extent and nature of the influence of heredity on the morbidity pattern of a population. Most diseases attributed to genetic defects are relatively rare with such diseases accounting for a small proportion of overall morbidity. At the same time, almost all diseases have a genetic component, with the importance of that component varying from disease to disease. Disorders where genetics play an important role, so-called genetic diseases, can be classified as single-gene (monogenetic) defects, chromosomal disorders, or multifactorial conditions. Mitochondrial disorders are a result of gene mutations.

Single-Gene (Monogenic) Disorders

A single-gene disorder is one that is determined by a single genetic locus and the specific allele on one or both members of a chromosome pair. Single-gene defects are rare, with a frequency of less than 1 in 200 births. But since there are about 6000 known single-gene disorders, their combined impact is significant. Single-gene disorders are characterized by a pattern of transmission within families, although monogenic disorders are relatively rare in comparison with more commonly occurring diseases, such as diabetes and heart disease.

Known single-gene disorders include the following:

Autosomal Recessive Genes

- ADA deficiency
- Alpha-1-antitrypsin deficiency
- Cystic fibrosis
- Phenylketonuria
- Sickle cell anemia
- Tay–Sachs disease

X-Linked Recessive Genes

- Duchenne muscular dystrophy
- Hemophilia A

Autosomal Dominant Genes

- Familial hypercholesterolemia
- Huntington's disease

Chromosomal Disorders

In chromosomal disorders, the defect is due to an excess or lack of the genes contained in a whole chromosome or chromosome segment. Chromosomal disorders include:

- Down syndrome
- Klinefelter syndrome
- Turner syndrome

(continued)

Exhibit 6.1 (continued)

Multifactor Disorders

Multifactorial inheritance disorders are caused by a combination of small inherited variations in genes, often acting together with environmental factors. Heart disease, diabetes, and most cancers are examples of such disorders. Behavioral disorders are also multifactorial, involving multiple genes that are affected by a variety of other factors. The genetic contribution to behavioral disorders such as alcoholism, obesity, mental illness, and Alzheimer's disease is increasingly being recognized. Multifactorial disorders include:

- Cancer
- Coronary heart disease
- Hypertension
- Stroke
- Obesity

Mitochondrial DNA-linked disorders

Mitochondrial disorders include more than 60 hereditary disorders that have been shown to result from changes (mutations) in mitochondrial DNA. Because mitochondria come only from the female egg, most mitochondria-related disorders are passed down only from the mother. Mitochondrial disorders can appear at any age and exhibit a wide variety of symptoms and signs. These disorders include:

- Blindness
- Developmental delay
- Gastrointestinal problems
- Hearing loss
- Heart rhythm problems
- Diabetes
- Neuropathy (including dementia)
- Epilepsy

Genetic factors are likely to play some role in high blood pressure, heart disease, and other vascular conditions. However, it is also likely that people with a family history of heart disease share common environments and risk factors that increase their susceptibility. The risk for heart disease can increase even more when heredity is combined with unhealthy lifestyle choices, such as tobacco use and poor dietary habits. Ultimately, it is believed that genetics accounts for less than 10 % of the morbidity found within the US population.

Biological Pathogens

Diseases arising from biological pathogens in the environment have been a constant companion of human populations. These pathogens take a variety of forms and have been responsible for the bulk of morbidity and mortality throughout human history. Most of these pathogens occur naturally in the environment, originating for the most part with animals. Many pathogens can adapt to a changing environment and through natural selection mutate and survive.

While most infectious diseases have been eliminated if not eradicated in modern developed countries, the threat of biological pathogens cannot be entirely removed. Despite extraordinary advances in the management of such diseases, the ease of world travel and increased global interdependence assure the continued impact of such conditions. Public health authorities in the US must constantly monitor disease trends in order to detect the emergence of new communicable diseases and the re-emergence of old ones. The most salient modern example of an emerging infectious disease is HIV/AIDS, which likely emerged a century ago after the virus jumped from one primate host to another and, as a result of a complex array of social and demographic factors, spread readily within the human population.

Biological pathogens have become less important in contemporary societies over time, accounting for as little as 10 % of the observed morbidity. Biological pathogens are grouped into the following categories:

Viruses

A viral disease (or viral infection) occurs when an organism's body is invaded by pathogenic viruses. Pathogenic viruses are mainly those of the families of: *Adenoviridae*, *Picornaviridae*, *Herpesviridae*, *Hepadnaviridae*, *Flaviviridae*, *Retroviridae*, *Orthomyxoviridae*, *Paramyxoviridae*, *Papovaviridae*, *Polyomavirus*, *Rhabdoviridae*, and *Togaviridae*. Some notable pathogenic viruses cause smallpox, influenza, mumps, measles, chickenpox, ebola, and rubella.

Bacteria

Although most bacteria are harmless and often beneficial, several are pathogenic. One of the bacterial diseases with the highest disease burden is tuberculosis, caused by the bacterium *Mycobacterium tuberculosis*, which kills about two million people a year. Pathogenic bacteria contribute to other globally important diseases, such as pneumonia and foodborne illnesses caused by bacteria such as *Shigella*, *Campylobacter*, and *Salmonella*. Pathogenic bacteria also cause infections such as tetanus, typhoid fever, diphtheria, syphilis, and leprosy. During the last decade, scientists discovered many new organisms and new strains of many familiar bacteria, such as *Escherichia coli*.

Fungi

Pathogenic fungi are fungi that cause disease in humans or other organisms. Although fungi are eukaryotic organisms, many pathogenic fungi are also microorganisms. Life-threatening fungal infections in humans most often occur in immunocompromised patients or vulnerable people with a weakened immune system, although fungi contribute to common problems among immunocompetent populations such as skin, nail, or yeast infections. The frequency of invasive, opportunistic fungi has increased significantly over the past two decades. This increase in infection is associated with excessive morbidity and mortality and is directly related to the increasing numbers of patients who are at risk for the development of serious fungal infections, including patients undergoing blood and marrow transplantation (BMT), solid-organ transplantation, and major surgery (especially gastrointestinal surgery); patients with AIDS, neoplastic disease, and advanced age; patients receiving immunosuppressive therapy; and premature infants.

Other Parasites

Human parasites include various protozoa and worms which may infect humans, causing parasitic diseases. Human parasites are divided into endoparasites, which cause infection inside the body, and ectoparasites, which cause infection superficially within the skin. The cysts and eggs of endoparasites may be found in feces, providing a means for the parasitic species to exit the current host and enter other hosts. Some eukaryotic organisms, such as protists and helminths, cause disease. One of the best known diseases caused by protists is malaria.

Prions

A prion refers to a protein-engendered infection, thus the conflation of "protein" and "infection". Prions are not considered as living organisms because they are misfolded protein molecules which may propagate by transmitting a misfolded protein state. If a prion enters a healthy organism, it induces existing, properly folded proteins to convert into the misfolded prion form. While several yeast proteins have been identified as having prionogenic properties, the first prion protein was discovered in mammals and is referred to as the major prion protein. Prions are abnormal proteins whose presence causes some diseases such as scrapie, bovine spongiform encephalopathy (mad cow disease), and Creutzfeldt–Jakob disease.

Animal Pathogens

Animal pathogens are disease-causing agents of wild and domestic animal species, at times including humans. Diseases spread by insects also fall into this category, with ticks and mosquitos being common carriers. Examples of diseases resulting from animal pathogens include rabies, plague, histoplasmosis, e. coli and Lyme disease. Animal pathogens are particularly common in regions where people live and/or work in close proximity to animals. In fact, 75 % of new infectious diseases that have emerged in the past ten years originated with animals. Vulnerable populations (e.g., young children, elderly, immunocompromised individuals) are particularly susceptible.

Environmental Factors

In epidemiology, an environmental disease is a disorder caused by factors in the physical environment and/or, increasingly, the social environment. Diseases that are not transmitted genetically or via infection are typically considered environmental diseases. It may, however, be more appropriate to refer to them as environment-engendered disorders. Although the morbidity patterns of all societies everywhere have been affected by their environments (after all, biological pathogens are part of the environment), the impact of the physical and social environments has emerged in modern society as a major contributor to the nature and level of morbidity within a population. The environmental threats faced by traditional societies appear insignificant in the light of the pervasive impact of modern society on our air, water, and soil.

Environmental factors can impact morbidity in a number of ways. The most obvious type of impact would be direct contact with an environmental toxin. This could involve contact with the skin or respiratory intake. Examples of diseases caused by physical factors in the environment include skin cancer caused by excessive exposure to ultraviolet radiation in sunlight and diseases caused by exposure to chemicals in the environment such as toxic metals.

Although direct contact certainly represents a health threat, a much greater threat involves in indirect influence of environmental factors. This would involve transmission of toxins through other often routine means. Thus, people ingest toxins through the water they drink, the food they eat, and through the second-hand smoke they inhale. Eating, drinking, and breathing are obviously routine activities that in a polluted environment put health at risk. Cancer acquired through breathing secondary smoke is a leading example, as are diseases caused by contaminated foods.

Another indirect means of environmental impact on health involves health risks fostered through the pollution of water and soil. Threats in the external environment include air pollution, soil and water contamination from arsenic, lead, benzene, mercury, and other toxic chemicals, and the side-effects of the use of fungicides and herbicides, insecticides, and pesticides. Natural and man-made disasters constitute environmental threats as well, not just from the direct effects of the disaster (e.g., direct exposure to toxic chemicals) but from the after-effects that might include air, soil, or water contamination and the psychological impact on those affected by the disaster. In the aftermath of a hurricane, for example, the water, soil, and even the air may be contaminated with pathogens that were not present—or at least not active—prior to the disaster. Thus, diseases such as cholera that had been previously contained may opportunistically reassert themselves. Even short of a natural disaster, a body of water that has been polluted by toxic waste becomes a breeding ground for a range of health risks.

Recent research has suggested that a less dramatic aspect of the environment—the weather—may be a predictor if not a contributor to morbid conditions (Strobe 2013). "Disease forecasters" have for some time been testing the feasibility of using weather forecasts to predict the outbreak of certain diseases. Using information on rain and snow and on patterns of plant growth among other factors, health officials have attempted to predict outbreaks of hantavirus, cholera, Rift Valley fever (in Africa), and influenza. An increase in respiratory conditions has been reported in the US over the past several years, particularly among children. It has been argued that polluted air weakens the system and opens the door for a variety of conditions related to respiration. Changes occurring in the world's climate are affecting our health and well-being, and will have even greater consequences in the future. (Exhibit 6.2 describes the potential impact of climate change on human health.)

It is felt that environmental factors may interact with genetic traits to trigger certain diseases that had previously been latent. In fact, there is a growing list of genetic diseases whose onset is thought to be initiated by environmental insults. These include cancer, diabetes, and heart disease among others. (If a disease process is concluded to be the result of a combination of genetic and environmental factor influences, its etiological pattern can be referred to as multifactorial.)

Although the risks of developing chronic diseases are attributed to both genetic and environmental factors, a much higher proportion of disease risks is probably due to differences in environments. The evidence shows that environmental risk factors play at least some role in more than 80 % of the diseases regularly reported by the World Health Organization. Globally, nearly one quarter of all deaths and the total disease burden can be attributed to the environment. In children, however, environmental risk factors can account for slightly more than one-third of the disease burden. (World Health Organization 2006).

While threats in the outdoor environment are likely to be top of mind, for many people environmental threats found indoors, particularly in the home, constitute a greater health risk. The latter include molds and other allergy producing pathogens, carbon monoxide and other toxic gases, second-hand smoke, and various physical conditions of housing (e.g., unsafe structural conditions, asbestos, lead, and formaldehyde in building materials). Many household products, it is now revealed, include potentially toxic chemicals. Exposure to toxins, pathogens, radiation, and chemicals found in almost all personal-care products and household cleaners are common environmental factors that contribute to a significant portion of non-hereditary diseases.

Exhibit 6.2 Climate Change and Morbidity

Scientists and health professionals have become increasingly concerned over the potential health implications of climate change. While much of the presumed impact has been speculative, there is a growing body of evidence of the impact that rising temperatures and abnormal weather patterns are already having on the morbidity patterns of the world's populations. This has led some to suggest that climate change represents the future's greatest public health threat.

According to the federal government's National Institute of Environmental Health Sciences, climate change is expected to affect morbidity through its impact on the following conditions:

Asthma, respiratory allergies, and airways diseases. Respiratory allergies and diseases may become more prevalent because of increased human exposure to pollen (due to altered growing seasons), molds (from extreme or more frequent precipitation), air pollution, and aerosolized marine toxins (due to increased temperature, coastal runoff, and humidity), and dust (from droughts).

Cancer. Many potential direct effects of climate change on cancer risk are anticipated, such as increased duration and intensity of ultraviolet radiation and exposure to toxic chemicals that are spread through floods and other natural disasters. Increase in ultraviolet radiation has implications both externally (e.g., skin cancer) and internally (e.g., immune system impact).

Cardiovascular disease and stroke. Climate change may exacerbate existing cardiovascular disease by increasing heat stress, increasing the body burden of airborne particulates, and changing the distribution of zoonotic vectors that cause infectious diseases linked with cardiovascular disease.

Foodborne diseases and nutrition. Climate change may be associated with staple food shortages, malnutrition, and food contamination (of seafood from chemical contaminants, biotoxins, and pathogenic microbes) and crops (by pesticides).

Heat-related morbidity and mortality. Heat-related illness and deaths are likely to increase in response to climate change. Heat-related events are already the most common cause of weather-related deaths, and climate change could contribute to increases in health exhaustion, cramps, heat stroke, and heat-related mortality.

Human developmental effects. Climate change is expected to affect normal human development in two major ways: malnutrition—particularly during the prenatal period and early childhood—as a result of decreased food supplies, exposure to toxic contaminants resulting from extreme weather events, increased pesticide use for food production, and increases in harmful algal blooms in recreational areas.

(continued)

Exhibit 6.2 (continued)

Mental health and stress-related disorders. By causing or contributing to extreme weather events, climate change may result in geographic displacement of populations, damage to property, loss of loved ones, and chronic stress. Posttraumatic stress disorders inevitably increase in the wake of extreme weather events.

Neurological diseases and disorders. Climate change, as well as attempts to mitigate and adapt to it, may increase the number neurological diseases and disorders in humans. Increases in the prevalence of neurological diseases (e.g., Alzheimer's disease and Parkinson's disease) are attributed in part to exposure to environmental risks.

Vectorborne and zoonotic diseases. Disease risk may increase as a result of climate change due to related expansions in vector ranges of animals and insects, shortening of pathogen incubation periods, and disruption and relocation of large human populations.

Waterborne diseases. Increases in water temperature, precipitation frequency and severity, evaporation–transpiration rates, and changes in coastal ecosystem health could increase the incidence of water contamination with harmful pathogens and chemicals.

Weather-related morbidity and mortality. Increases in the incidence and intensity of extreme weather events such as hurricanes, floods, droughts, and wildfires may adversely affect people's health in direct and indirect ways during and following the event.

Source: National Institute of Environmental Health Sciences

Increasing attention is being paid to the impact of the social environment on morbidity patterns. Environments that are characterized by insecurity, threats to physical safety, and a lack of basic resources contribute to the onset of illness, the progression of disease, and potentially unfavorable outcomes for both physical and mental disorders. A growing body of evidence points to the role of stress in the emergence of a wide range of health conditions. Stress plays a direct role in the onset of various emotional and psychiatric conditions and is known to trigger certain physical illnesses (e.g., asthma, arthritis). (Additional implications of the social environment are discussed below with regard to lifestyles.) Exhibit 6.3 describes the role of stress in the onset of disease.

Clearly the environment is impinging on the health of the population in various direct and indirect ways and growing in significance. The estimate by the WHO that environmental factors account for 24 % of the total contribution to morbidity should probably be considered conservative, with this likely to increase due to ongoing environmental insults and, now, the impact of climate change. A recent massive study of morbidity patterns in the US and worldwide adjudged air pollution to be one of the top 10 risk factors for disability (Murray et al. 2013).

Exhibit 6.3 Stress and Morbidity

Stress is a normal psychological and physical reaction to positive or negative situations faced by living organisms, including human beings. Stress itself is not abnormal nor necessarily detrimental but has the potential for both positive and negative effects. The body responds to stress in various ways. Adrenaline generated by stress increases the heart rate, elevates the blood pressure, and boosts energy supplies. Cortisol, the primary stress hormone, increases sugars (glucose) in the bloodstream, enhances the brain's use of glucose, and increases the availability of substances that repair tissues. Cortisol also curbs functions that would be nonessential or detrimental in a fight-or-flight situation. It alters immune system responses and suppresses the digestive system, the reproductive system, and growth processes. Cortisol levels are increasingly used to measure stress, and research has tied elevated cortisol levels to a number of health conditions.

Stress becomes an issue with regard to physical or mental health when it exceeds the body's normal coping capacity. If stress makes it difficult to carry out one's daily routine, an adjustment disorder may develop. When one's mind and/or body are constantly on edge because of excessive life stress, serious health problems may result. Stress can affect hormonal and immune system functions with detrimental effects on the lining of arteries. It can cause the production of fibrinogen which can cause blood clots. The fact that some people get sick and others do not, may ultimately reflect their ability to handle stress.

There is ongoing debate over the importance of the various forms that stress takes, particularly the difference in impact on the body between chronic everyday stress and a traumatic event. Both types of stress can impact an individual, but the burden of everyday stressful life circumstances is more relevant for the study of morbidity. Studies are emerging that suggest that many of the differences in the observed onset of physical and mental disorders and variations in the progression of disease, clinical outcomes, and even mortality rates are a function of differences in the level of chronic stress, all other factors being equal. Thus, research on differences in clinical outcomes for whites and blacks when acuity levels and treatment modality are controlled suggests that the observed differences reflect a lifetime of unremitting stress on the part of the latter (Mancino et al. 2001).

Based on self-reported health status measures, respondents who report themselves to be in only fair or poor health also report higher levels of stress. They are also more likely to report physical symptoms of stress than thoseExhibit 6.3 (continued)who rate their health as excellent or very good. Measures

(continued)

Exhibit 6.3 (continued)

of perceived stress also correlate with higher levels of physical and mental morbidity.

The typical diet of the US population contributes to stress in a very direct manner. High sugar content foods in particular affect the body by inducing an immediate "high" followed by a slower but nevertheless impactful decline in metabolism. Both the rapid increase and rapid decrease in blood sugar levels create friction within the body, with this stress accompanied by increased blood pressure and a higher heart rate. Friction that is frequent within the organism creates wear and tear on the body. Many of the so-called diseases of civilization (e.g., heart disease, diabetes, arthritis) are ultimately caused by this type of mechanical friction.

The following health conditions (among others) are thought to be triggered or exacerbated by stress:

- Obesity
- Heart disease
- High blood pressure
- Abnormal heart beat
- Asthma
- Menstrual problems
- Acne and other skin problems
- Digestive problems
- Various mental disorders
- Impaired memory
- Sleep disorders

Lifestyles

As US morbidity patterns have evolved, increasing attention has been paid to the role of lifestyles in the level and nature of morbidity. "Lifestyles", simply put, refers to patterns of behavior or the way of life characterizing a population. (References are made to an individual's "lifestyle" but it is group patterns of living that are of interest to demographers.) A group's lifestyle reflects a combination of tangible and intangible factors. Tangible factors involve the demographic variables associated with individuals or groups, whereas intangible factors concern the psychological aspects of group members such as personal values, preferences, and outlooks. A lifestyle typically reflects the attitudes, values, and worldview of members of a particular group. A group's lifestyle provides a means of forging a sense of self for the group member and includes the cultural symbols that resonate with personal identity. While individual lifestyles are sometimes considered voluntary, members of various groups tend to have their attitudes and behaviors shaped and ultimately constrained by group norms.

The diseases that have come to be dominant within the US population are increasingly referred to as "diseases of civilization," reflecting the notion that our "civilized" way of life is contributing to our health problems. These diseases appear to increase in frequency as countries become more industrialized and more people live to old age. These diseases include Alzheimer's disease, atherosclerosis, asthma, cancer, chronic liver disease and cirrhosis, chronic obstructive pulmonary disease, type 2 diabetes, heart disease, metabolic syndrome, Crohn's disease, nephritis and chronic renal failure, osteoporosis, stroke, depression, obesity, and sexually transmitted infections.

Diet, physical activity, adiposity, alcohol consumption, and cigarette smoking have all been associated with increased risk of chronic diseases including type 2 diabetes, cardiovascular diseases, and various cancers (van Dam et al. 2008). In fact, the prevalence of type 2 diabetes, hypertension, arthritis, and some cancers for Americans who are overweight or obese has more than doubled during the last 40 years. As a result, over 50 % of premature deaths in Western countries can be attributed to lifestyle. Non-communicable diseases such as cancer, cardiovascular disease, and diabetes account for 35 million deaths worldwide each year or 60 % of all deaths. These diseases typically exhibit the following risk factors: tobacco use, inappropriate diet, and physical inactivity (World Health Organization 2009).

One study (van Dam et al. 2008) found that the probabilities of death from a variety of causes was considerably lower for those who avoided the five most common lifestyle risk factors. They found the risk of mortality in the presence of lifestyle risks was 4.31 times greater for all causes, 3.26 greater for cancer, and 8.17 greater for cardiovascular disease. A total of 28 % of deaths during the 24-year follow-up period could be attributed to smoking and 55 % to the combination of smoking, being overweight, lack of physical activity, and a low diet quality.

Some of the lifestyle factors reflect the routine activities characterizing the lives of individual citizens. These include dietary habits, exercise patterns, sleep adequacy, and even the use of automobile seatbelts. The first three are clearly linked to obesity which in turn is linked to a variety of diseases of civilization. A massive study of disease trends in the US and worldwide found diet to account for the greatest part of differences in morbidity. Differences in diet were found to account for 26 % of deaths and 14 % of disability-adjusted life-years (Murray et al. 2013). Other significant contributors to morbidity and disability were tobacco use (second) and obesity (third). Interestingly, high cholesterol actually was found to have declined as a factor in differential morbidity. (Exhibit 6.4 discusses the link between obesity and morbidity.)

Exhibit 6.4 Obesity and Morbidity

The trend toward increased levels of obesity within the US population has raised concerns among health professionals over its long-term impact on morbidity. The terms "overweight" and "obesity" refer to body weight that is greater than what is considered healthy for a certain height. People classified as "obese" have an abnormally high and unhealthy proportion of body fat. Obesity is considered a morbid condition in its own right but is also associated with a wide range of other health conditions. The following disorders are considered to be caused, triggered, or exacerbated by obesity.

Coronary Heart Disease

As one's body mass index rises, so does the risk of coronary heart disease (CHD). CHD is a condition in which plaque builds up inside the arteries that supply oxygen-rich blood to the heart. Plaque can narrow or block the coronary arteries and reduce blood flow to the heart muscle. This can cause angina or a heart attack. Obesity also can contribute to heart failure or the progressive deterioration of heart function.

High Blood Pressure

One's chances of having high blood pressure are greater if they are overweight or obese. If blood pressure rises and stays high over time, it can damage the body in a variety of ways.

Stroke

Being overweight or obese can lead to a buildup of plaque in the arteries. Eventually, an area of plaque can rupture, causing a blood clot to form. If the clot is close to the brain, it can block the flow of blood and oxygen to the brain and cause a stroke. The risk of having a stroke rises as BMI increases.

Type 2 Diabetes

In type 2 diabetes, an acquired form of the disease, the body's cells do not use insulin properly resulting in excessive sugar in the blood. Diabetes is a leading cause of early death in its own right but also contributes to the development of CHD, stroke, kidney disease, and blindness. Most people who have type 2 diabetes are overweight.

Cancer

Obesity is associated with increased risks for several types of cancer, including cancers of the esophagus, breast (postmenopausal), endometrium (the lining of the uterus), colon and rectum, kidney, pancreas, thyroid, gallbladder, and, potentially, cancers affecting other sites. The percentage of cancer cases attributed to obesity varies widely for different cancer types but is as high as 40 % for some cancers.

(continued)

Exhibit 6.4 (continued)

Osteosarthritis

Osteoarthritis is a common joint problem of the knees, hips, and lower back. The condition occurs if the tissue that protects the joints wears away. Extra weight can put more pressure and wear on joints, thereby triggering osteoarthritis.

Sleep Apnea

Sleep apnea is a common disorder in which a person has one or more pauses in breathing or shallow breaths during sleep. One cause of sleep apnea is excess fat stored around the neck. This can narrow the airway, making it hard to breathe.

Obesity Hypoventilation Syndrome

Obesity hypoventilation syndrome (OHS) is a breathing disorder that affects some obese people. In OHS, poor breathing results in too much carbon dioxide (hypoventilation) and too little oxygen in the blood (hypoxemia). OHS can lead to serious health problems and may even cause death.

Reproductive Problems

Obesity is associated with several reproductive disturbances. Whereas mechanisms by which obesity affects fertility are complex and still not completely understood, obesity affects the body's metabolism and chemical balance. Increasing evidence points to the long-term impact of early onset (childhood/adolescence) obesity as a predictor of infertility. Obesity is also a contributor to menstrual disorders.

Gallstones

People who are overweight or obese are at increased risk of producing gallstones. In addition, being overweight may result in an enlarged, poorly functioning gallbladder.

In addition to the above, it is now realized that overweight and obesity also increase the health risks for children and teens. Type 2 diabetes, for example, once was rare in American children, but an increasing number of children are developing the disease today. Also, overweight children are more likely to become overweight or obese as adults, increasing the disease risks noted above.

Source: National Heart, Lung and Blood Institute (2013). *What Are the Health Risks of Overweight and Obesity?* Downloaded from URL: http://www.nhlbi.nih.gov/health/health-topics/topics/obe/risks.html.

Another category of risk involves clearly dangerous behaviors. This would include binge drinking, reckless driving, and risky sexual behavior. The combination of alcohol and a number of other factors represents a potentially explosive cocktail that carries some risk of short-time health threats and certain risk of long-term health implications.

Some aspects of lifestyle relate more directly to the matter of health behavior ("healthstyles"). With the emergence of the fitness craze in the 1970s and various wellness movements since, the notion of a lifestyle built around health and wellness evolved. An emphasis on preventive health measures, for example, could be considered a lifestyle attribute. Other practices—regular physical and dental checkups, compliance with one's medical regimen, appropriate use of prescription drugs—are lifestyle-related behaviors that have implications for morbidity.

Lifestyle (or psychographic) analysis is commonly used in consumer product and service industries and has been applied to a limited extent to healthcare. The rationale for using lifestyle analysis is based on evidence that demographic characteristics alone cannot explain variations in morbidity or predict health behavior. It has been found, for example, that some groups with similar demographic attributes actually display quite different lifestyles.

In an attempt to quantify lifestyle differences, a variety of psychographic classification systems have been developed. The intent is to segment the population in terms of its lifestyle attributes, and this is typically accomplished by profiling the population with regard to a number of relevant variables, segmenting the population based on the clustering of attributes, and assigning an appropriate label to the psychographic cluster.

Once a psychographic cluster is established it becomes possible to (1) assign clusters to any group or even any household and (2) associate a wide range of characteristics with that cluster. Thus, if a household or group is assigned to the "Pools and Patios" cluster it is possible to determine its characteristics in terms of age, race/ethnicity, income and educational level, and community type among others. More important, however, is the ability to profile the target group in terms of various lifestyle attributes—consumer behaviors, exercise patterns, recreational activities, dietary preferences, and so forth—that might contribute to morbidity.

Although health professionals have been slow to associate health-related variables with psychographic clusters, an increasing amount of information has become available in this regard. More obvious applications are the association of alcohol and drug abuse and various mental disorders with certain lifestyle groups. Even more common conditions, however, can often be associated with specific lifestyle clusters. Patterns of distribution for diabetes, asthma, and heart disease, along with various disabilities, for example, correlate with psychographic patterns. An example where psychographics trump demographics might be in the case of heart disease—where two populations may display similar age and sex distributions but vary significantly in terms of both heart disease morbidity and mortality. While lifestyles might not account for all of the difference, evidence suggests that lifelong patterns of diet, exercise and tobacco and alcohol abuse—i.e., lifestyle attributes—are more significant than the importance of advanced age in shaping morbidity patterns.

One final point to be made concerning lifestyles relates to the discussion of demographic correlates of morbidity considered in the next chapter. As noted above, demographic attributes are incorporated into the development of lifestyle segmentation systems. While psychographics attempt to transcend the limitations of demographic analysis, there is an inherent demographic aspect to any psychographic classification system. Indeed, it could be argued that many psychographic differences identified actually reflect underlying demographic attributes. For that reason certain lifestyles may be associated with specific demographic groups. African-American teenagers, affluent housewives with young children ("soccer moms"), college students, and similar demographic groupings come to mind, with their lifestyle attributes tied very closely to their demographic roots. Further evidence of the psychographic/demographic link is provided when observed lifestyles change as demographic status (e.g., age, marital status, income level) changes. (Exhibit 6.5 discusses the role of lifestyles in morbidity.)

Medical Science

The contributions to morbidity discussed so far could be considered "passive" influences in that, for the most part, their impact on morbidity is unplanned and often unanticipated. (An exception would be the healthy lifestyle movement noted above.) In contrast, the *raison d'etre* for medical science is the modification of morbidity patterns and the reduction of mortality. From one perspective it could be argued that the level and nature of morbidity in contemporary US society is a function of the contribution that medical science has made in the control and/or eradication of various diseases. The fact that we do not suffer today, it could be argued, from polio, measles, or other communicable diseases is a reflection of the application of medical science. While this appears a plausible explanation for morbidity patterns, this conventional wisdom, as shown below, is not universally accepted.

Exhibit 6.5 Psychographic Segments and Morbidity

Lifestyle (or psychographic) analysis is commonly used in consumer product and service industries but has only been applied to a limited extent to healthcare. The rationale for using lifestyle analysis is based on evidence that demographic characteristics alone cannot explain variations in morbidity or predict health behavior. It has been found, for example, that some groups with similar demographic attributes actually displayed quite different lifestyles.

A good case in point might be the analysis of the health service needs of Medicaid enrollees, particularly with the prospect of increases in enrollment in the Medicaid program under the Affordable Care Act. In order to qualify

(continued)

Exhibit 6.5 (continued)

for this federal-state healthcare program for low-income individuals, income and personal assets have to fall below a certain level. Further, up until the changes proposed under the Affordable Care Act, participation was essentially limited to mothers and their children. These constraints would suggest that Medicaid enrollees would essentially fall into the same lifestyle cluster. However, when an analysis was completed using the Mosaic segmentation system which, at the time, involved 60 different lifestyle clusters, it was found that Medicaid enrollees could be found in at least 8 of the 60 clusters. Thus, Medicaid enrollees included inner-city minority populations (probably the stereotypical cluster), rural Appalachian clusters, small town clusters, and residents of Indian reservations among others. Far from representing a homogeneous grouping of poor people, Medicaid enrollees represented a number of different subgroups. Of significance for morbidity analysis, these subgroups suffered from different types of health problems requiring custom health system solutions rather than a one-size-fits-all approach.

As a simple example of variations in morbidity by lifestyle, the following graphic illustrates differences in the rate of hypertension and diabetes for selected Mosaic psychographic clusters:

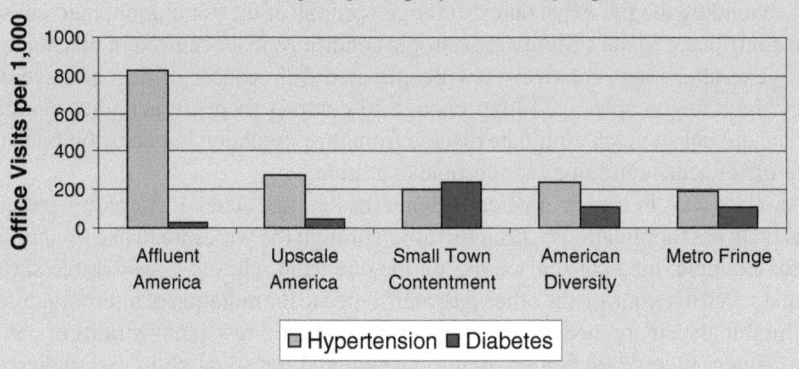

Numerous other examples of differences based on lifestyle can be offered. It is found for example that when populations of senior citizens are compared, some have higher rates of hospitalization for heart disease than others. Given that heart disease correlates closely with age, one would expect similar patterns of hospital use based on physiology if nothing else. However, the rate of hospital discharges for heart disease for the affluent elderly is much lower than that for poverty-level elderly. Since we are talking about populations

(continued)

Exhibit 6.5 (continued)

covered under the Medicare program, health insurance should not be a determining factor, leaving one to speculate as to the role of lifestyles in heart disease morbidity. Numerous examples can be provided of groups of patients with similar demographic characteristics who were provided similar health services for similar health problems but report quite different clinical outcomes, suggesting that the lifestyles of the respective patient groups are more of a determinant of outcomes than the actual care received.

Unquestionably, there are a number of ways in which the actions of medical practitioners contribute to the morbidity patterns that exist within the US population today. As noted above, the development of therapies, drugs and, in particular, immunizations to combat the communicable diseases that plagued the population until well into the twentieth century played a significant role in eliminating the epidemic diseases that accounted for the most of the morbidity (and mortality) at the beginning of that century.

These developments in medical science had the dual effect of eliminating certain diseases and laying the groundwork for the emergence of others. By eliminating the diseases that were common in childhood along with other acute conditions, and, thus, extending the life expectancy for large portions of the population, medical science contributed to the shift toward chronic conditions that occurred in that century. Four generations ago, relatively few people died from cancer or degenerative diseases since few people lived long enough to contract them. In actuality, medical science did not so much eliminate disease from the population but contributed to the trade-off of acute conditions for chronic conditions.

Another way in which medical science has contributed to morbidity patterns reflects its past application of drug therapy. Through the widespread use of antibiotics for example, medical science has on the one hand relieved considerable suffering and saved lives but, on the other, has contributed to the mutation of microorganisms resulting in the emergence of new—and often antibiotic-resistant—strains of pathogens. Again, it could be argued, that this amounted not so much to the eradication of disease but a swapping of one disease for another.

It should also be noted that the success of medical science has led to the emergence of additional health problems. A case in point would be medicine's ability to save the lives—and maintain viability—of individuals who would not have survived in previous eras. Through emergency and trauma care, many lives are saved and individuals are able to return to society. Similarly, modern technology can keep severely premature babies alive that would have died in the past. The downside of the intervention of medical science is the creation of a large number of disabled individuals who would not have survived in previous periods. This means that the number and proportion of the US population that is disabled are greater today than at any time in the past. This fact is not solely the consequence of the application of medical science, of course, but our society's ability to save lives and maintain viability has clearly been a contributor.

An additional argument for the role of medical science in contemporary morbidity patterns is the negative impact of the healthcare system itself on the health of the population. Conditions that are caused by the healthcare system—iatrogenic conditions—have become increasingly common. A leading example would be the proportion of hospital patients that contracts some condition while hospitalized other than the one for which they were admitted. Or the fact that accidental falls in hospitals are a major health consideration. Then there are the situations of missed diagnoses, inappropriate or inadequate treatment, or outright negligence on the part of healthcare providers. In addition to suffering from the side-effects of many therapies, particularly drug therapy, a large proportion of the population has become dependent on prescription drugs. While the therapeutic benefit of most drugs is not in dispute, the negative impact of "polypharmacy" is also indisputable, with addiction to prescription drugs becoming an increasingly common disorder.

One source of data on the level of adverse effects from the healthcare system can be found in a study by the Centers for Disease Control and Prevention (Bernstein et al. 2003). The study found that for 1999–2000 the rate of emergency department visits for adverse effects of treatment was 4.5/1000 for those under 65 years, 6.6/1000 for those 65–74 years, and 12.9/1000 for those 75 years and over. For hospital discharges attributable to adverse effects of treatment, the respective rates in 1999–2000 were 3.7/1000, 20.7/1000, and 31.0/1000, suggesting a significant level of hospital admission for treatment for the adverse effects from previous treatment.

Ultimately, a case can be made that, while medical science has had a significant impact on personal health, it has had much less impact on "population health" which, of course, is the focus of this book. The improvement in the health status of the population observed during the twentieth century can be primarily attributed to improved standards of living, better housing, better nutrition, and better public sanitation. To the extent that medical science played a role, it was primarily by means of the application of public health principles through which the health status of the population as a whole was improved, rather than through the application of medical science to individual members of society. Conventional wisdom now suggests that as little as 10 % of the variation in morbidity in contemporary society can be attributed to medical science. Exhibit 6.6 addresses the historic role of medical science in the nature of disease in US society.

Exhibit 6.6 What Happened to the Epidemics: Medical Science or Demographics?

During the twentieth century, the US, along with the rest of the world's developed nations, experienced a dramatic decline in mortality. From 1900 to the mid-1970s, the mortality rate (adjusted for age and sex) in the US dropped from nearly 17.5 per 1000 population to barely 5 per 1000. Over this period, a 69.2 % decrease in overall mortality was recorded, with most (92.3 %) of this occurring during the first 50 years of the twentieth century. It is likely that the decline in mortality, for some causes of death at least, actually commenced during the 1800s. Due to a lack of data, however, the "documented" decline in mortality is usually reported to have occurred during the first half of the twentieth century.

The most direct explanation for the decline in mortality is well documented. This period of history witnessed the virtual eradication of several of the contagious diseases that had been the leading causes of death since the Middle Ages. In the US in 1900, 40 % of the deaths were attributable to 11 major infectious conditions. These included measles, tuberculosis, pneumonia, diphtheria, scarlet fever, typhoid, influenza, whooping cough, poliomyelitis, smallpox, and diseases of the digestive system. By the mid-1970s, these conditions combined accounted for only 6 % of the nation's deaths. While death rates due to these conditions were dropping precipitously, little decline was seen in the rates for other non-contagious conditions. In fact, chronic conditions were dramatically increasing their share of the mortality rate.

The ultimate question becomes: What was responsible for the virtual elimination of these killer diseases during the first half of the twentieth century? This question is conventionally answered by pointing to breakthroughs on the part of medical science that led to the eradication of these diseases. Many cite this period as the conclusive proof for the efficacy of medical science in dealing with these nearly universal health threats. Medical science has perpetuated the notion that its efforts in the development of cures for these killers were the primary factors in reducing their threat to the population. The general public has accepted this argument and become a willing supporter for this explanation of the elimination of epidemic diseases.

An increasing number of researchers in both Europe and the US, however, have argued that medical science has had a limited impact on these killer diseases and, therefore, has made little contribution to the reduced mortality experienced since 1900. While conceding that some major breakthroughs occurred during the late 1800s and early 1900s in terms of our understanding of the causes and cures of these epidemic diseases, it is argued that factors other than medical care were responsible for the dramatic drop in mortality.

(continued)

McKinlay and McKinlay (1977) contend, after examining the relationship between mortality trends and developments in medical science, that the timing of the development of "cures" for these conditions virtually eliminates them as an explanation for the recorded reduction in mortality. The McKinlays argue that, for the ten infectious conditions for which there is adequate information available, the therapeutic agents developed to counteract them were introduced long after declines in mortality had begun occurring. For example, by the time a vaccine had been developed in 1943 to combat influenza, this condition had virtually ceased to be a significant cause of death. In fact, 75 % of the decline in mortality from influenza between 1900 and 1973 had occurred by the time the vaccine was introduced in 1943.

Similar scenarios can be constructed for most of the other major infectious diseases. It is further noted that most of the reduction in mortality in the US overall occurred prior to 1950—that is, before expenditures for health services reached an appreciable level. The McKinlays contend that "3.5 % probably represents a reasonable upper-limit estimate of the total contribution of medical measures to the decline of mortality in the US since 1900" (McKinlay and McKinlay 1977, p. 425).

If medical science cannot be credited with the elimination of these epidemic diseases, what can? There is now widespread support for the notion that changes in the sociocultural characteristics of the population, rather than medical care, accounted for the bulk of the mortality decline documented. Changes in the political, economic, and social environment in the US had brought about changes in the demographic structure of the population. There had been a general improvement in socioeconomic conditions and educational levels, as well as improvements in nutrition. A similar pattern of social change characterized industrialized European countries as well.

McKeown et al. (1972) concluded that the decline in mortality in several European countries during the second half of the nineteenth century was attributable to rising standards of living (especially improvements in diet), improvements in hygiene, and a healthier environment. Therapy, it was argued, made virtually no contribution to this improvement. Dubos (1959) argued convincingly for nonmedical—primarily demographic—explanations for the decline in mortality, and Fuchs (1974) clearly implicates rising incomes, not medical technology, in the reduction in mortality, beginning in the middle of the nineteenth century.

While conventional beliefs concerning the elimination of the epidemic diseases are still maintained by many within medical circles and among the general public, by the 1970s the research emphasis had substantially shifted away from its focus on the medical factors involved in the reduction of morbidity and mortality. The importance of demographic and sociocultural characteristics as factors associated with the nation's morbidity patterns and mortality levels has now become widely recognized.

(continued)

Exhibit 6.6 (continued)

References

Dubos, R. J. (1959). *Mirage of health*: *Utopias*, *progress and biological change*. New Brunswick, NJ: Rutgers University Press.
Dubos, R. (1965). *Man adapting*. New Haven, CT: Yale University Press.
Fuchs, V. R. (1974). *Who shall live*? New York: Basic Books.
McKeown, T., Brown, R. G., & Record R. G. (1972). An interpretation of the modern rise of population in Europe. *Population Studies 9*, 119–141.
McKinlay, J. B., & McKinlay, S. J. (1977). The questionable contribution of medical measures to the decline of mortality in the United States in the twentieth century. *Milbank Memorial Fund Quarterly/Health and Society* (Summer), 405–428.

Clearly, a number of factors contribute to the morbidity patterns observed for the US population. The various factors considered here along with the demographic contributors discussed in the next chapter suggest a complex set of factors influencing the pattern of morbidity observed at any point in time. McGinnis et al. (2002) attempted to determine the relative contribution made by various factors to a population's morbidity configuration. Although somewhat dated, their conclusions described in Exhibit 6.7 are still considered relevant today.

Exhibit 6.7 The Leading Determinants of Health

For at least 20 years the changing nature of the factors that contribute to the health and illness characterizing a given population have been debated. Just as the diseases that affect the US population have changed over the past century, the factors that contribute to observed morbidity patterns have also changed. McGinnis et al. (2002) have provided a summary (up to that date at least) of the various contributions that different factors make to the amount and nature of ill-health within the population. They envision these factors in five domains.

Genetics is certainly a factor in the health status of the population. Although genetic diseases account for a negligible proportion of deaths, gene defects account for a wide variety of health conditions and may account for up to 60 % of late onset diseases such as diabetes and heart disease. Due to the large number of diseases that have some genetic component, the authors estimate that 30 % of health conditions can be attributed to heredity.

A population's "social circumstances" has been increasingly cited as a determinant of health and illness. Health is influenced by education, employment, income disparities, poverty, housing, crime, and social cohesion. Throughout the life cycle, the social circumstances that affect individuals contribute to their lifestyles and life chances, and exposure to various social factors is likely to affect the status of individuals many years after the fact. Poverty by itself is thought to account for 60 % of mortality and presumably a similar or greater amount of morbidity. The ubiquitous nature of social

(continued)

circumstances caused the authors to indicate that they account for 15 % of the observed differences in health status.

In considering the impact of environmental factors, the authors include biological pathogens (microbial agents) with hazards in the form of toxic agents (e.g., air/water pollution, occupational products) and structures hazards (e.g., worksite conditions, home hazards). Microbial agents have become less significant as other aspects of the environment have come to the fore. Environmental factors are thought to account for 5 % of the observed differences in health status.

According to McGinnis, Williams-Russo, and Knickman, behavior patterns represent the most dominant domain of influence over health status today. Referred to elsewhere as "lifestyles," the authors point out the far-reaching influence of patterns of diet, exercise, and social behavior. The things that we do to ourselves—what we choose to eat, how much physical activity we participate in and what we do for recreation, for example—all affect our health status. This domain includes the positive steps we take—adequate sleep, use of automobile seatbelts, preventive checkups—and the negative influences that we avoid (or not)—alcohol, tobacco and drug abuse, risky sexual behavior. These factors taken together are thought to account for fully 40 % of the observed differences in health status.

The authors cite the various commentators noted early on the limited impact that medical care actually exerted on the morbidity pattern of our society. While medical care certainly benefits individual patients and available treatments and technology contribute to overall health status to some extent, these benefits are to a certain extent nullified by the negative impact of medical care on people's health. The Centers for Disease Control and Prevention (CDC) have consistently placed the impact of medical care on our population's health at around 10 %.

The graphic below illustrates the distribution of domain influence from the perspective of the authors:

Factors Influencing Health Status

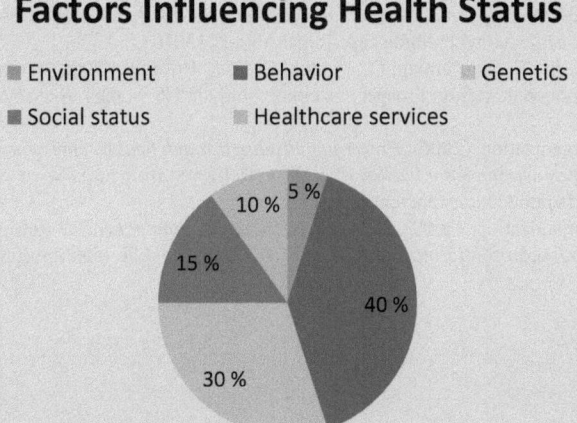

■ Environment   ■ Behavior   ■ Genetics

■ Social status   ■ Healthcare services

(continued)

Exhibit 6.7 (continued)

Source: McGinnis, J.M., Williams-Russo, P., and J.R. Knickman (2002). The Case for More Active Policy Attention to Health Promotion. *Health Affairs* 21(2):78–93.

References

Bernstein, A. B., Hing, E., Moss, A. J., Allen, K. F., Siller, A. B., & Tiggle, R. B. (2003). *Health care in America: Trends in utilization*. Hyattsville, MD: National Center for Health Statistics.

Dubos, R. J. (1959). *Mirage of health: Utopias, progress and biological change*. New Brunswick, NJ: Rutgers University Press.

Dubos, R. (1965). *Man adapting*. New Haven, CT: Yale University Press.

Fuchs, V. R. (1974). *Who shall live?* New York: Basic Books.

Mancino, A. T., Rubio, I. T., Henry-Tillman, R., et al. (2001). Racial differences in breast cancer survival: The effect of residual disease. *Journal of Surgical Research, 100*(2), 161–5.

McGinnis, J. M., Williams-Russo, P., & Knickman, J. R. (2002). The case for more active policy attention to health promotion. *Health Affairs, 21*(2), 78–93.

McKeown, T., Brown, R. G., & Record, R. G. (1972). An interpretation of the modern rise of population in Europe. *Population Studies, 9*, 119–141.

McKinlay, J. B., & McKinlay, S. M. (1977). The questionable contribution of medical measures to the decline of mortality in the United States in the twentieth century. *Milbank Memorial Fund Quarterly/Health and Society, 55*(3), 405–428.

Murray, C. J. L, Abraham, J., Ali, M. K., et al. (2013). The state of US health: 1990–2010: Burden of diseases, injuries and risk factors. *Journal of the American Medical Association*. Retrieved from http://jama.jamanetwork.com/article.aspx?articleid=1710486&utm_source.

National Genome Research Institute. (2013). Frequently asked questions about genetic diseases. Retrieved from http://www.genome.gov/19016930.

National Institute of Environmental Health Sciences. (2013). Gene-environment interaction. Retrieved from http://www.niehs.nih.gov/health/topics/science/gene-env/.

National Heart, Lung and Blood Institute. (2013). *What are the health risks of overweight and obesity?* Retrieved from http://www.nhlbi.nih.gov/health/health-topics/topics/obe/risks.html.

Strobe, M. (2013). *Disease forecasters rely on weather forecast*. Associated Press. Retrieved from http://www.weather.com/health/disease-forecasters-20130103.

van Dam, R. M., Li, T., Spiegelman, D., Franco, O. F., & Hu, F. B. (2008). Combined impact of lifestyle factors on mortality: Prospective cohort study in US women. *British Medical Journal, 337*, a1440.

World Health Organization. (2006). *Preventing disease through healthy environments: Towards an estimate of the environmental burden of disease*. Retrieved from http://www.who.int/quantifying_ehimpacts/publications/preventingdisease/en/.

World Health Organization. (2009). *Do lifestyle changes improve health?* Retrieved from http://www.who.int/mediacentre/multimedia/podcasts/2009/lifestyle-interventions-20090109/en/index.html.

Additional Resources

Bullard, R. (2000). *Dumping in Dixie: Race, class, and environmental quality* (3rd ed.). Boulder, CO: Westview Press.

National Institute for Allergy and Infectious Disease. (2012). *Bacterial infections*. Retrieved from http://www.niaid.nih.gov/topics/bacterialinfections/pages/default.aspx.

Nature Publishing Group (Periodical). *Emerging microbes and infections*. On-line journal.

Oxford University Press (Periodical). *Journal of Infectious Diseases*.

Chapter 7
Demographic Factors Associated with Morbidity

Introduction

The impact of demographic attributes on morbidity patterns is being increasingly recognized by health professionals and demographers. There is a growing body of evidence on the correlation between various demographic traits and health status, with some even ascribing causation to certain demographic characteristics. Further, an analysis of demographic attributes provides insights into the manner in which morbidity in general and in its specific forms is distributed within the population. Because this book is targeted toward demographers, the demographic correlates of morbidity are accorded a separate chapter.

Examining the factors affecting the morbidity of the population as a whole often masks important differences that exist among subgroups. It is not unusual to have a figure for a county, for example, that reports an average rate when virtually no subpopulation actually exhibits that rate. In Shelby County, Tennessee, in 2005 the county-wide infant mortality rate was 13 per 1000 live births. What this rate doesn't tell us, however, is that the figure for African-Americans is 19 per 1000 and that for whites is 6 per 1000. For that reason it is important to decompose these figures and examine subsets of the population under study based on race, sex, age, or some other attribute relevant under the circumstances.

It is also important to examine morbidity for segments of the population that reflect a combination of different variables. For example, when levels of morbidity for various conditions are examined, the study population is often broken down into the race/sex categories of white males, white females, black males, and black females, with the differences between the subgroups examined. This allows for a

© Springer New York 2016
R.K. Thomas, *In Sickness and In Health*, Applied Demography Series 6,
DOI 10.1007/978-1-4939-3423-2_7

more in-depth appreciation of the morbidity indicator under study and should be a prerequisite for anyone seeking to understand an indicator's significance within that population.

One other issue when considering the demographic correlates of health and illness is the potential interrelationship of the variables in question. While demographic attributes are addressed separately in the sections that follow, the likelihood of interaction between the attributes being considered needs to be kept in mind. An obvious example is the well-known relationship between education and income, but there are other potential interactions as well (e.g., race and income, occupational status, and education). While every possible interaction cannot be addressed in this chapter, readers should remain sensitive to the possibility of the interaction of demographic variables with one another.

Biosocial Characteristics

Biosocial characteristics are so called because they are attributes that are rooted in biology but also have a social dimension. These attributes include age, sex, race, and ethnicity. While age and sex represent biological states, social attributes are ascribed to persons of different ages and a social dimension (i.e., masculinity and femininity) is associated with the respective sexes. Race is not a scientific category but exists as a social construct, thus displaying both biological and social dimensions. Ethnicity refers to one's cultural heritage and is not a clearly biological state. However, to the extent that ethnic groups tend to interbreed and maintain a distinct gene pool, ethnicity is included in the biosocial category. Note that biosocial characteristics are ascribed at birth and are not amenable to change. Exhibit 7.1 presents data on some of the demographic correlates of morbidity as represented by health status.

Age

There has been long-standing acceptance of the notion that morbidity patterns are linked closely with age. Conventional wisdom suggests that as a person ages, health problems become more numerous and more serious. While there is some truth to this assertion, research conducted in recent years indicates that the situation is more complex than had been previously thought. Patterns of morbidity, disability, and even mortality display complicated relationships with the age structure of the population.

As one would expect, positive self-assessment of health declines as people age. While about 74 % of those aged 15–44 describe their health as excellent or very good, only 33 % of those 75 and over feel the same way (National Center for Health Statistics 2012). The association between age and self-assessed health status is complicated in that some research has found that health status assessment among older Americans can actually improve over time.

The conventional wisdom that the number of health problems increases as the population ages is a somewhat misleading notion. Although it is true that the prevalence of *chronic* conditions does increase with age, and there appears to be a clear cumulative effect, the incidence of *acute* conditions actually declines with age. Thus, while the younger age cohorts are characterized by high rates of respiratory conditions, injuries, and other acute conditions, the elderly are relatively free of these. Instead, they face a growing number of chronic conditions such as hypertension, arthritis, and cancer. It has been suggested that the average *number* of conditions does not differ much from the youngest age cohorts to the oldest. The differential is primarily in the types of conditions common to the various age cohorts and in the severity of those conditions (National Center for Health Statistics 2012).

There is a well-documented relationship between the prevalence of mental illness and age, although the nature of the relationship has undergone substantial modification in recent years. Until the 1970s, it was believed that aging had a cumulative effect on mental health just as it did on physical health (U.S. Department of Health and Human Services 1999a, b), with the prevalence of mental illness thought to increase with advancing age. However, many observers argued that this pattern reflected selectivity in terms of the mental disorders measured, use of statistics on institutionalized patients, and the tendency to attribute many symptoms of old age to mental illness. In terms of observed cumulative prevalence of mental disorders, in fact, those 30–44 years exhibit the highest rate (55.0 %) while those 60 years and older the lowest (26.1 %). The 18–29-year-old cohort records a rate of 52.4 %, almost as high as the 30–44 year group, while the 45–59 age cohort records a rate of 46.5 % (Kessler, Berglund, Demler et al. 2003).

Figures from this same study indicate that the age of greatest mental illness risk is a function of the type of disorder. Depression, for example, is more common among those 18–25 years and least common among those 50 years and older (with an average age of onset of 23 years). Similarly, those 18–29 years exhibit the highest rates of bipolar disorder, those 30–44 years the highest rate for anxiety disorders and obsessive compulsive disorders, and those 45–59 years the highest rate for post traumatic stress disorders. For essentially every mental disorder examined, the elderly exhibited the lowest rate.

These figures suggest a non-monotonic and much more irregular relationship, primarily reflecting a rethinking of the conditions classified as mental disorders. The inclusion of alcoholism, drug abuse, and suicide under the heading of mental illness has created a "morbidity bulge" in the 15–25 age cohort. At the same time, attributing many symptoms of aging to Alzheimer's disease has reduced the perceived prevalence of mental illness among the elderly. Further, the advent of adolescent treatment centers has meant that many more adolescents are being defined as mentally disturbed than in the past (Maughan et al. 2005).

Not surprisingly, there is a clear correlation between age and the level of disability characterizing a population. The proportion of the population experiencing some level of activity limitation increases steadily with age, and the oldest age cohorts are characterized by limited-activity days several times as numerous as those for younger age cohorts. For example, 6 % of the 15–44 age cohort in 2010 reported *some* limitation of activity. The comparable figure for the 65–74 age group was over 26 % (National Center for Health Statistics 2011). Similarly, data from the 2011 American Community Survey indicate a steady increase in the level of disability from the youngest age cohort to the oldest (5.1 % for youth and 50.7 % for those 75 and older).

The most well-established relationship has been the association between age and mortality, with mortality sometimes used as a proxy for morbidity. Overall, there is a direct and positive relationship between age and mortality in contemporary US society. The 2007 age-specific mortality rate of 15/100000 for those aged 5–14, the cohort with the lowest rate, increases gradually up through age 50. After age 50, the increase in the mortality rate is dramatic (National Center for Health Statistics 2010a, b).

More important from a morbidity analysis perspective the causes of death vary widely among the age cohorts. For example, the leading causes of death for infants (under 1 year) are birth defects, respiratory conditions, and infectious diseases. The leading causes for young adults are accidents and suicide; for young adult African-Americans homicide is added to the list. The elderly are more likely to fall victim to the major killers: heart disease, cancer, and stroke. Ultimately, each age cohort has its own peculiar cause-of-death configuration. To a certain extent these differences in mortality patterns reflect differences in morbidity patterns. However, the emergence of chronic diseases has complicated the relationship between morbidity and mortality in that chronic diseases are not necessarily the direct cause of death.

Sex

One of the most perplexing but important associations discussed in this context is that between sex and morbidity. There is perhaps no other demographic variable for which differentials in health status are so clear-cut. Yet, at the same time, there is probably none for which more questions are raised concerning the meaning of the findings and the possible explanations for observed relationships.

Any discussion of the relationship between sex and health status must begin with what has become a maxim: Women are characterized by higher levels of morbidity than men, but men have a higher mortality rate. Although this is a somewhat simplistic summary of a complex situation, there is a great deal of evidence to suggest that, by any measure of morbidity one would care to use, women are "sicker." On the other hand, there is no doubt that mortality rates are higher and life expectancy is lower for males in contemporary US society (Rogers et al. 2000).

When global measures are utilized, females tend to characterize themselves as being in slightly poorer health than males (National Center for Health Statistics 2012). The difference in perceived health status is narrow (males are slightly more positive), and much of the variance is probably explained by the older age structure of the female population. On more specific measures, however, females tend to score much higher (i.e., they report more symptoms). For virtually all reported conditions and diagnoses, females are characterized by higher incidence rates (National Center for Health Statistics 2012).

When the prevalence of chronic diseases is reviewed, it is found that males report higher rates of heart disease (e.g., coronary heart disease, hypertension), although the rate for strokes is similar for males and females (National Center for Health Statistics 2012). On the other hand, females report higher rates for respiratory conditions (e.g., asthma, chronic bronchitis) although males and females report similar rates for emphysema. Women account for virtually all cases of breast cancer and men for all cases of prostate cancer. Arthritis is more common among women as are migraines and severe headaches. While females report an even higher level of chronic conditions than acute conditions, these tend to be conditions that are not life-threatening. Although males are sick less often and report fewer symptoms, when men do become ill the condition is likely to be more serious or even fatal.

The relationship between sex and mental health status is fairly well documented, although the conclusions are not without controversy. Based on reported symptoms, clinical evaluations by community researchers, and frequency of presenting themselves for mental healthcare, females appear to be characterized by a higher level of mental disorder. Women are more likely to report frequent feelings of sadness, with this condition reported by 14 % of women and 10 % of men. Women also report higher levels of nervousness and restlessness (National Center for Health Statistics 2012). Women exhibit higher scores on indices of depression, hysteria, and paranoia as well as on less severe mental disorders, but men exhibit a greater prevalence of antisocial disorders, authority problems, and Type A behavior (World Health Organization, N.D.). In the major national study conducted on psychiatry morbidity, women were 70 % more likely to experience a major depressive disorder (Kessler et al. 2003). This same study, however, concluded that there was little difference in the lifetime prevalence between men and women when all disorders are considered.

As with physical disorders, females tend to be characterized by milder, more common conditions such as neuroses. Males, on the other hand, tend to be characterized by more serious psychoses. A major exception is found in the case of depression, for which women report a rate twice as high as men (World Health Organization, N.D.). As with physical illness, it appears that females are characterized by a greater occurrence of symptoms while males are afflicted with more extreme conditions.

It is beyond the scope of this book to evaluate the various explanations that are offered to account for these phenomena. There is evidence that women are more sensitive to the existence of symptoms of both physical and mental illness, that they are more willing to admit or report their symptoms, and that they more readily take action in response to perceived symptoms, thereby showing up more often when morbidity data are compiled (Gijsbers van Wijk and Kolk 1997). And, of course, in US society it is more culturally acceptable for women to be ill.

Many observers suggest that females are not, in fact, "crazier," but that differences in identified prevalence rates are a function of other factors (Eaton et al. 2011). These factors include a tendency for females to perceive symptoms as emotional rather than physical, the greater tendency for females to admit to symptoms of either kind, and the willingness of society to interpret females' characteristics as emotional rather than physical.

Exhibit 7.1 Self-Assessed Health Status for Adults by Selected Biosocial Characteristics, US, 2010

Characteristic	Excellent (%)	Very good (%)	Good (%)	Fair (%)	Poor (%)
Total	36.0	30.4	23.9	7.4	2.2
Age					
Under 12 years	55.7	27.2	15.2	1.8	0.1
12–17 years	53.8	26.7	17.3	2.0	0.3
18–44 years	37.4	33.1	23.2	5.3	1.0
45–64 years	23.7	31.4	28.9	11.6	4.4
65–74 years	16.6	29.7	32.5	16.0	5.1
75 years and over	11.6	24.5	35.5	30.6	7.7
Sex					
Male	36.7	30.4	23.7	7.0	2.2
Female	35.3	30.4	24.2	7.8	2.3
Race/ethnicity					
White	37.6	30.9	22.7	6.8	2.1
Black	27.7	36.8	30.5	11.6	3.3
Asian	36.3	30.8	24.8	6.6	1.6
American Indian	22.7	31.7	27.6	13.6	4.4
Hispanic	30.8	27.7	28.5	10.4	2.7

Source: National Center for Health Statistics (2011). *Summary health statistics for the U.S. Population*: *National Health Interview Survey, 2010*. Bethesda, MD: National Center for Health Statistics

Males, while scoring "better" on the indicators of morbidity discussed above, are at greater risk of mortality. In effect, the age-adjusted mortality rate for males is slightly higher than that of females, with males recording a mortality rate of 8.2 per 1000 in 2011 compared to 6.3 per 1000 for females. For each of the 15 leading causes of death in 2007, males recorded a higher mortality rate, and for three causes the male/female ratio was over 3:1 (Xu et al. 2010). The mortality rate for males is in fact higher at every age. Indeed, the death rate for males is even higher than that for females during the prenatal period, indicating that the greater mortality risk characterizing males predates birth. At ages 15–24 and 35–44, the mortality rate for males is almost three times as high. The differential in sex-specific mortality rates translates into differential life expectancy, with females born in 2010 expected to live 81.0 years on the average compared to a life expectancy of 76.2 years for males (National Center for Health Statistics 2013).

For every condition except diabetes and sex-related disorders, the mortality rate is higher for males. A major killer of infants is chronic respiratory disease, a condition more common among male infants. Accidents are the major cause of death for children aged 1–14, with males having approximately twice the risk of accidents. Homicide is a major cause of mortality for those 15–25, with males accounting for most of the homicide deaths. Similar patterns can be found for subsequent age cohorts and other health conditions (National Center for Health Statistics 2010a, b).

With regard to disability, comparable proportions of males and females are characterized by some level of activity limitation. The 2012 National Health Interview Survey found 18 % of females and 13 % of males to exhibit at least one physical disability. Females, however, accumulate on the average more work-loss days, more school-loss days, and more bed-restricted days (National Center for Health Statistics 2012). Women reported an average of six bed-days per year related to some disability compared to 4 bed-days for men.

Race/Ethnicity

Racial groups are defined based on one or more distinguishable physical attributes considered important in the particular society. Race is a clearly biosocial attribute, because it combines physical attributes with social connotations. In US society and many others, skin color is the most important factor in racial categorization. The racial categories used by the US Census Bureau and applied here include: whites (or Caucasians), blacks (or African-Americans), Asian and Pacific Islanders (or Asian-Americans), American Indians, and other. (The Census Bureau also recognizes individuals of two or more races but there is as yet limited morbidity data on that racial category.)

Ethnic group distinctions are based on differences in cultural heritage rather than physical characteristics. Members of distinct ethnic groups have a common cultural tradition, including values and norms and perhaps even a language that sets them apart from the larger society. While ethnic distinctions are not primarily biological, prolonged "inbreeding" often leads to the development of distinctive physical characteristics. For this reason the discussion of ethnicity and morbidity is included in this section. The major ethnic groups in US society include Hispanics, Jews, and certain large national groups that, in some regions at least, have been able to maintain their ethnic identity. The only "official" ethnic group recognized by the Census Bureau is "Hispanics."

When the various racial groups in the US are examined in terms of morbidity patterns, significant differences are found. The major distinction is between whites and blacks, with Asian-Americans and American Indians manifesting less distinct morbidity characteristics (National Center for Health Statistics 2011). The discrepancy by race (blacks are less positive) is substantial, however, with African-Americans reporting much less favorable health conditions than whites. Given that blacks have a younger age structure, the true differential is even larger than observed disparities. While only 8.7 % of whites assessed their health as fair or poor in 2009, the figure was 14.2 % for blacks, despite a younger age structure. Differences in self-assessed health status should be interpreted with caution, however, since there are indications that members of different racial groups may use different criteria for assessing their own health status (Brandon and Proctor 2010).

Clear-cut differences in morbidity are found primarily between whites and African-Americans. The number of symptoms, the number of illness episodes, and the severity of the conditions all place African-Americans at a morbidity disadvantage. Although relatively more prone to acute health conditions, African-Americans actually suffer higher rates of both acute and chronic conditions than whites. African-Americans represent 12 % of the population, for example, but account for 28 % of the diagnosed hypertension (Lloyd-Jones et al. 2010). The morbidity disadvantage for African-Americans is reflected in the proportion over-weight or obese, with a rate of 69 % recorded for this group compared to 54 % for whites (Mead et al. 2008). Further, all things being equal, African-Americans contracting life-threatening conditions are more at risk of death than are whites with the same condition (See, for example, American Lung Association 2011). Even at higher income levels, African-Americans still report higher levels of chronic disease than comparable whites.

Differences in cause-specific morbidity exist between various racial and ethnic groups, with the epidemiology of cancer reflecting this phenomenon. Whites in the US are more likely to suffer from colon/rectal cancer, breast cancer, and bladder cancer, for example, than are African-Americans. On the other hand, the incidence of lung, prostate, stomach, and esophageal cancer is higher for African-Americans. Asian-Americans are less likely to suffer from heart disease than either whites or African-Americans, and even Hispanics record lower age-adjusted rates of heart disease than non-Hispanic whites. Both Asian-Americans and Hispanics report lower rates of respiratory diseases than non-Hispanic whites (National Center for Health Statistics 2012). The prevalence rate for HIV/AIDS for African-Americans is ten times that for whites (Mead et al. 2008). Although much of the black/white disparity is attributed to socioeconomic status differences, Sims et al. (2011) found that, after adjustment for age, gender, and socioeconomic status, a lifetime of stress and the burden of discrimination were associated with greater hypertension prevalence.

Specific ethnic groups are similarly likely to display unique cancer morbidity profiles. Polish-Americans suffer from relatively high levels of lung and esophageal cancer, for example, while among Italian-Americans bladder, intestinal, and pharyngeal cancer are more common. Japanese-Americans suffer from stomach cancer at rates many times higher than Japanese nationals, while cervical cancer is almost unknown among Jewish women. (See, for example, Seeff and McKenna 2003.)

The distribution of mental illness with regard to race and ethnicity has been of great interest to researchers and health professionals. Historically, it was believed that blacks and certain other racial and ethnic groups in US society were character-ized by worse mental health status than whites. Even after the scientific study of mental illness became established, evidence was developed that suggested higher rates of mental disorder among these non-white groups. African-Americans were most often singled out and depicted as a group as being disproportionately characterized by psychotic disorders.

Researchers now believe that the impression of higher rates of mental disorder among blacks and certain other racial and ethnic groups is a function of at least three factors: (a) collection of data historically from public mental institutions; (b) a middle-class bias in the diagnosis of mental disorders; and (c) a failure to consider important intervening variables such as social class (Murali and Oyebode 2004). Current research suggests that differences in types of mental pathology make comparisons based on race problematic (Riolo et al. 2005).

The major national study on psychiatric morbidity (Kessler et al. 2003) found that African-Americans were 30 % *less* likely to experience *any* mental disorder over their lifetimes compared to whites. To the extent that differences do exist, the disparity appears to be not in prevalence but in types of disorders. Blacks seem to be characterized by more severe forms of disorders (e.g., psychoses), and whites by milder forms (e.g., neuroses), although this same study indicated that blacks were 40 % less likely to experience a major depression disorder over their lifetimes.

The relationship between mental disorder and ethnicity is even cloudier, given the wide variation in the types of ethnic groups in US society. Some groups, such as Mexican-Americans, appear to be characterized by higher than average rates of disorder (U.S. Department of Health and Human Services 1999a, b). Others, such as Japanese- and Chinese-Americans, appear to be relatively "disease-free" (Meyers 2006). Once again, the observed differences may be a reflection of socioeconomic differences or even migration status. In any case, it is extremely difficult to compare subgroups of the population in terms of either prevalence or types of mental disorders due to numerous possible intervening variables.

Indicators of disability are found to be higher among African-Americans than among other racial groups. Data from the 2010 National Health Interview Survey indicated that 12.2 % of the white population had some limitations due to disability, compared to 16.5 % of the African-American population (National Center for Health Statistics 2011). In addition, African-Americans are characterized by higher levels of disability than whites, whether measured by the actual presence of handicaps or by such proxy measures as work-loss days and bed-restricted days. This disability disparity for African-Americans exists at even high income levels. The disability rate for Hispanics is one-third lower than the average.

Mortality rates for the black population are considerably higher than those for the white population. When mortality rates are examined for 2011, the overall mor-tality rate for the US population is 7.4 per 1000 population. The age-adjusted mor-tality rate for the white population as a whole was 7.4 deaths per 1000 population, compared to 8.8 per 1000 population for blacks (National Center for Health

Statistics 2010a, b). Age-adjusted mortality rates for other groups in 2011 were 5.4 for Hispanics, 6.0 for American Indians, and 4.1 for Asian-Americans. African-Americans are characterized by higher mortality risks at nearly all ages and for nearly all causes (Rogers et al. 2000). (Note that all of these rates are age-adjusted, thereby eliminating any distortion caused by differentials in age distribution.)

Further, important differences exist between blacks and whites in terms of the common causes of death, and to a great extent these differentials reflect differences in morbidity characteristics. Whites in the US are more likely to die from chronic conditions, especially those associated with aging. Blacks and members of certain ethnic groups are relatively more likely to die from acute conditions. Further, non-whites are more likely to be affected by environmentally caused health problems and life-threatening problems associated with lifestyles (such as homicide, HIV/AIDS, and accidents). Consequently, the dominant causes of death among the white population are heart disease, cancer, and stroke. African-Americans, on the other hand, are more likely to die as a result of infectious conditions, respiratory and digestive systems conditions, and the lifestyle-associated problems noted above. Mortality disparities for some health conditions actually exceed the morbidity disparity. For example, African-American men report a 50 % higher prevalence rate for prostate cancer but a 100 % higher mortality rate from this condition than do white males.

Much of the mortality advantage characterizing Asian-Americans and Hispanics has been attributed to the foreign-born among these populations. Subsequent generations of Asian-Americans and Hispanics, it seems, do not fare as well in comparative mortality analyses. Interestingly, Native Americans have made the greatest gains of any group in reducing mortality in recent years, with an age-adjusted mortality rate in 2011 of 6.0 per 1000 (National Center for Health Statistics 2010a, b). Native Americans record the lowest mortality for cancer of any group but by far the highest mortality rates for diabetes, suicide, and accidents.

Another relatively important cause of death for blacks is infant mortality. Although infant mortality was dramatically reduced as a cause of death in the US during the last century, it continues to be a serious health threat for non-whites. The infant mortality rate for African-Americans in 2011 was more than twice that for whites, 11.4 per 1000 live births versus 5.1 (Hoyert and Xu 2012). The rates for both groups have declined since the late 1980s, with the gap between the two actually narrowing in recent years.

Other racial and ethnic groups recorded quite disparate rates of infant death. Certain Asian-American groups, for example, report much lower than average infant mortality, while Hispanics as a group record infant mortality rates between those of whites and blacks. Native Americans and native Alaskans historically have recorded very high infant mortality rates; however, since the 1950s, their rates have come to resemble the US average. Infant mortality rates for selected groups in 2009 were 5.3 for Hispanics, 8.5 for American Indians, and 4.4 for Asian-Americans (Mathews and MacDorman 2013). The Hispanic infant mortality rate is something of an anomaly, given the relatively poor health status of this population and this group's lower level of access to health services. The low Hispanic infant mortality rate is generally attributed to the emphasis on family within this culture.

Sociocultural Characteristics

Sociocultural characteristics refer to traits exhibited by individuals that refer to their position or status in society. While biosocial traits are essentially ascribed at birth, sociocultural traits are typically acquired through the actions of the individual. Sociocultural traits are important not only because they indicate one's place in society, but because of their contribution to the morbidity patterns of the population.

Marital Status

Early on in the study of demographic influences on morbidity, it was concluded that marital status was a predictor of both health status and health behavior (Verbrugge 1979), although (as will be shown) the relationship is a highly compli-cated one. The categories of marital status for the discussion below will be: never married, married, divorced, and widowed. (The term "single" has generally been eliminated from research terminology since it can be interpreted to mean never married, widowed, or divorced.) By the mid-1980s, most researchers counted couples living together as married. Separated individuals are not treated in a consistent manner in the literature but are most often listed under their official status, which is married. Some studies, however, list these couples as divorced if they are legally separated. This group is small enough however that this "married but separated" category does not distort the relationships identified by researchers.

Married individuals are found to have lower levels of morbidity and to perceive themselves as being in much better health than their unmarried counter-parts. Married persons also report a higher level of physical and psychological well-being than those who are not married (Shoenborn 2004). Further, it has been found that married individuals, when affected by a health condition, experience less serious episodes, face more favorable prognoses, and report more favorable outcomes than unmarried individuals facing the same condition. For some conditions, however, the never married are better off than the married (National Center for Health Statistics 2012).

These patterns hold, incidentally, for every age cohort. In fact, the advantage for the married increases with age for some conditions. While the prevalence of chronic conditions for the married and never married is approximately the same for the 18–24 age cohort, the NHIS found that one-third of the never married in the 45–64 age group suffer from chronic disabilities, compared to one-fifth of the ever married.

A notable exception to these patterns relates to the incidence of acute conditions and certain chronic conditions. Married men and women report slightly more acute conditions than never married men and women. However, the married are still better off overall than the divorced and widowed. It has been suggested that the never

married may suffer fewer episodes of acute conditions but are affected by more serious and prolonged conditions. It may be the case that married persons are more likely
to have their acute conditions diagnosed in a timely fashion. The incidence of injuries also represents something of an exception; while married people are less prone
to injuries than never-married and divorced individuals, they are more at risk for
injuries than are the widowed (National Center for Health Statistics 2012).

The preponderance of research now indicates that the different marital statuses
are at varying risks of mental illness. The 2009 NHIS found, for example, that 3.5 %
of the married reported chronic nervousness, a much lower figure that that for the
never married (5.1 %), the divorced (6.6 %), or the widowed (11.9 %). While the
married appear to be much better off overall in terms of mental health than are those
in any of the other marital categories, there is less consensus concerning the relative
risk for mental disorders for the never married, the divorced, and the widowed.
When mental health is measured in terms of feelings of sadness, hopelessness, and
worthlessness, the married report the lowest rates across the board. The never
married report the second lowest rates with the widowed and divorced exhibiting
much higher rates than either of these two groups (National Center for Health
Statistics 2012).

Evidence for the importance of marital status as a predictor of morbidity levels
can be drawn from data on changes in health status that accompany changes in marital status. When individuals shift from one status to another, changes in morbidity
are frequently seen. The observed negative trend is greatest when the shift is from
the married to the divorced or widowed category (Aseltine and Kessler 1993).

Such a general overview tends to mask a number of variations not apparent
when the overall pattern is examined. If figures for the various categories are
decomposed on the basis of other variables and if specific health problems
are considered, substantial variation is indicated by the data. For example, while
married individuals are healthier overall and married females are in relatively
good physical health, married females have been found to account for a large
amount of reported depression. Similarly, married males are better off than the
unmarried in general, but are likely to have higher mortality rates than never-
married females. In fact, married males are the ones found to suffer the most
deterioration (both physically and mentally) in making the transition from
married to unmarried statuses.

With regard to disability, only 13 % of married people were found to have
physical limitations in the 2009 National Health Interview Survey, compared to
15 % or more for those in other marital status categories. The pattern is similar with
regard to other indicators of disability. However, the NHIS found that married individuals report more work-loss days per year (3.4) compared to the never-married
(2.8 %), but less than the 5.4 days reported for the divorced and 6.0 days for the
widowed (Pleis et al. 2010).

As for many of the demographic variables discussed, the relationship may not
be as direct as it appears. There are those that argue for marital status-specific
disorders and others that contend that reliance on marital categories overlooks

differences between sexes. Another school of thought suggests that it is not marital status per se that correlates with risk of mental disorder but living arrangements. That is, those living alone (regardless of marital status) are at greater risk of mental disorder than those living with a significant other (Australian Bureau of Statistics 1997).

Income

Income is the measure of socioeconomic status that is most frequently linked to morbidity. It has been found that no matter what indicator is utilized, there is generally an inverse relationship between income and level of morbidity for both physical and mental disorders. As income increases, the prevalence of both acute and chronic conditions decreases. When symptom checklists are utilized, the lower the income the larger the number of symptoms identified. Not surprisingly, members of lower-income groups assess themselves as being in poorer health than do the more affluent. While 21.8 % of those living at or below the poverty level considered themselves in poor or fair health, only 4.3 % of those with household incomes four times the poverty level (i.e., $100000 or more) reported poor or fair health (National Center for Health Statistics 2011).

The levels of both acute and chronic conditions increase as income decreases. Morbidity differences based on income are particularly distinct for chronic conditions. For the lowest income group (those with household incomes less than $35000) the prevalence rate for heart disease in 2011 was 14 % compared to 10 % for those in the highest income group (those with household incomes of $100000 or more). Similar disparities are noted for diabetes (11 % vs. 6 %), emphysema (3 % vs. 1 %), kidney disease (3 % vs. 1 %), and arthritis (25 % vs. 19 %). An exception is found in the case of cancer, wherein the highest income group reports a rate of 9 % compared to 7 % for the lowest income group (National Center for Health Statistics 2012). Higher rates are also recorded among the lowest income groups for most chronic respiratory conditions. Note that, if the lowest income group is broken further (e.g., into <$15000, $15000–$24999, etc.), the disparities exhibited would be even greater at the lowest income levels.

Not only are there more episodes of certain types of both acute and chronic conditions recorded as income decreases, but the severity of the conditions is likely to be greater when income is lower. When afflicted by acute conditions, the poor tend to have more prolonged episodes characterized by greater severity. Interestingly, in a society that has become characterized by chronic health conditions, acute disorders remain surprisingly common among the lower income groups. In fact, the disease profile of many low-income communities more closely resembles that of a less developed nation than it does the US. It has also been found that living in poverty in childhood can have detrimental health effects later in life (Evans and Kim 2007). Interestingly, the relationship between income and health status remains even in the face of improved health behaviors on the part of the lower income groups (Lantz et al. 1998).

Early on in the study of the social epidemiology of mental disorder, it was asserted that the lower classes were more prone to psychiatric pathology than the affluent (Hollingshead and Redlich 1958). However, more recent studies have failed to consistently support this contention. What has been demonstrated is the fact that the relative prevalence of mental illness by social class depends heavily on the type of disorder examined. Further, for some disorders apparent correlations with other variables (e.g., race and age) are moderated when socioeconomic status is controlled (Mossakowski 2008). A more recent study (Jitender et al. 2011) found a direct relationship between income levels and psychiatric symptoms, with the number of DSM indicators increasing with decreasing income.

Although the possibility of diagnostic bias is always present, the preponderance of evidence indicates that different disorders characterize those at different socioeconomic levels. Further, those at the lower income levels are likely to be characterized by more severe disorders. This explains why early studies concluded that mental disorders were concentrated within lower-income groups; the available statistics were for schizophrenia cases recorded at public mental hospitals. It is still felt that schizophrenia, certain forms of depression, and sociopathy are more common among lower income groups. Manic-depression and neuroses, on the other hand, appear to be more common among upper income groups. The rate of suicide, it should be noted, is much higher for the affluent than for the non-affluent.

There is also an inverse relationship between income and indicators of disability. Among the population with annual household incomes in 2010 less than $35000, 20.6 % reported some limitation of activity due to chronic conditions. This figure drops dramatically to 8.9 % for the $35000–49999 income group. The rate continues to drop to a level of only 6.6 % for those with household incomes of $100000 or more (National Center for Health Statistics 2011). When examined in terms of poverty status, it is found that 28 % of the poor report disabilities, compared to 22 % of the near-poor, and 12 % of the non-poor. Further, the lower the income, the greater the number of bed-disability days, work-loss days, school-loss days, and restricted activity days reported.

The mortality rate for the lowest income group is considerably higher than that of the most affluent, even after adjusting for age (Rogers et al. 2000). The poor are also characterized by relatively high levels of infant mortality and even maternal mortality. Virtually all infant mortality in the US today is accounted for by the lowest income groups, and maternal mortality (which has been virtually eliminated society-wide), is disturbingly common among the poor and appears to be increasing.

One factor associated with income level is access to health insurance. In fact, access to health insurance is increasingly considered a predictor of morbidity. Exhibit 7.2 discusses the relationship between access to health insurance and morbidity.

Exhibit 7.2 Health Insurance Coverage and Health Status

The US is unique among modern, industrialized nations with regard to the financing of health services for its citizens. Most similar countries have national healthcare systems with a single mechanism (usually taxes) through which individuals pay for the healthcare they receive. Although in the US, the government does play a role in the financing of healthcare, this is primarily through the Medicare and Medicaid programs (for the elderly and the indigent, respectively). For those not qualifying for Medicare or Medicaid, their primary option is commercial insurance (either through group or individual plans), often provided through one's place of employment. In recent years the proportion of US residents covered by employer-sponsored insurance has declined, while the proportion covered under government programs has increased.

A significant portion of the population is uninsured and, although addressed somewhat by the passage in 2010 of the Affordable Care Act, tens of millions of Americans still lack health insurance. Of those who do have insurance, almost one in five has two or more different types. The extent to which an individual or family has health insurance varies with the situation and is liable to change over time. It is not unusual for a patient to have his medical costs covered through some combination of sources (e.g., Medicare, Medicaid, and out-of-pocket payments). The table below indicates the estimated distribution of insurance coverage types for the US population in 2009 (based on the American Community Survey).

Insurance source	Percent (%)
Commercial insurance	60
Medicare	10
Medicaid	13
Other federal insurance[a]	2
Uninsured	15

[a]Military insurance, Veterans Administration, other federal

Data generated through the National Health Interview Survey indicate a correlation between the type of insurance coverage and health status (National Center for Health Statistics 2011). For those under 65 years of age, 4.1 % of those with private insurance reported poor or fair health status, compared to 22.3 % of those on Medicaid. Only 9.8 % of the uninsured considered themselves in poor or fair health, no doubt reflecting the fact that many young adults are uninsured. Not surprisingly, 28.6 % of those 65+ (with Medicare coverage) reported poor or fair health status. Some 28.5 % of those on Medicaid reported limitations due to chronic disease,

(continued)

Exhibit 7.2 (continued)

compared to only 5.7 % of those with commercial insurance and 7.8 % of the uninsured. Again, not surprisingly, 33.2 % of those 65 and over and covered by Medicare report such limitations.

In terms of the prevalence of specific conditions, as above the major differences are between those with private insurance and those covered under Medicaid. Differences were found for example in the prevalence of diabetes (5.3 % vs. 12.3 %), kidney disease (0.7 % vs. 3.9 %), and arthritis (14.7 % vs. 23.7 %).

The relationship between presence of and type of health insurance and morbidity is a complicated one, and the nature of the relationship is not always clear. However, for our purposes it can be argued that type of insurance coverage is a reasonable predictor of health status in general and the prevalence of certain health problems in particular.

Education

The relationship between educational level and morbidity exhibits a similar pattern to that for income. Those at higher educational levels are likely to rate themselves as being in better health than those with less education (National Center for Health Statistics 2011). Over one-fourth (27.4 %) of those with less than high school educations report only poor or fair health status, compared to 15.8 % for those with a high school education and 6.2 % for those with a college degree. Similarly, the better educated report fewer episodes of acute conditions and chronic conditions than the poorly educated (National Center for Health Statistics 2012). The prevalence of heart disease (e.g., coronary heart disease, hypertension) increases as educational level decreases. The same pattern—higher rates with declining education holds—for chronic respiratory conditions, arthritis, and diabetes. The proportion of the population reporting diabetes, for example, decreases from 15 % for those with less than a high school education to 7 % for those with at least a bachelor's degree.

The relationship between educational level and mental illness, like that for physical illness, appears fairly clear-cut. In fact, some researchers have suggested that the income differentials noted above are in reality a function of differing levels of education. For example, adults with less than a high school education report the highest rates of sadness, hopelessness, and worthlessness while those with at least a bachelor's degree report the lowest rates. Further, the poorly educated are more likely to report feelings of nervousness and restlessness. As the level of education increases, there appears to be an increase in the prevalence but a decrease in the severity of disorders. The better educated appear to be more characterized by neurotic conditions, while the less educated appear to be more frequently psychotic. Ironically, the rate of suicide is much higher among the better educated.

The level of disability exhibits a clear pattern with regard to educational attainment. Research by the National Center for Health Statistics (2011) found that 25 % of those with less than a high school diploma reported difficulties with physical functioning, compared to 20 % of those with a high school diploma, 17 % of those with some college, and 10 % of those with at least a bachelor's degree. Further, adults with less than a high school education reported eight bed-days annually due to some disability, compared to three bed-days annually for the best educated. This is true for disability arising from both acute and chronic physical conditions. An analysis of data from the National Health Interview Survey found an inverse relationship between educational levels and chronic conditions, limitation of activities, and number of bed days for disability.

The pattern with regard to mortality also resembles that exhibited for income. The death rate for the poorly educated is much higher than for those with higher educational achievement (National Center for Health Statistics 2010a, b). According to NCHS data, the risk of mortality for those with a high school education is 60 % higher than that for those with a graduate degree (Rogers et al. 2000).

Like the poor, the causes of death for the poorly educated are more likely to be the acute problems associated with less developed countries than the chronic conditions characterizing much of American society. Also like the poor, the poorly educated are likely to be characterized by lifestyle-related deaths such as homicides and accidents. Education, in fact, has been shown to demonstrate a stronger association with mortality than income (Rogers et al. 2000).

Infant mortality, once a leading cause of death, has been virtually eliminated from the groups with the highest educational levels. The poorly educated as it turns out account for the bulk of infant deaths. The correlation between educational level and infant mortality rates is reflected in differences in low birth weight babies and premature births for those at different educational levels. Nine percent of mothers with less than a high school education deliver low birth weight babies, while this figure drops to 5.5 % for women with one or more years of college (National Center for Health Statistics 2010a, b).

As with income, the relationship does not necessarily reflect the level of education per se but the consequences of varying educational levels. Those with less education also are likely to have been more affected by financial insecurity, poor housing conditions, and unsafe environments, all contributing to an increase in morbidity levels. Exhibit 7.3 presents data on self-reported health status by selected sociocultural characteristics.

Exhibit 7.3 Self-Assessed Health Status for Adults by Selected Sociocultural Characteristics, US, 2010

Characteristic	Excellent (%)	Very good (%)	Good (%)	Fair (%)	Poor (%)
Total	36.0	30.4	23.9	7.4	2.2
Education					
Less than high school	15.6	22.1	34.8	19.9	7.5
High school diploma	21.6	30.1	32.5	12.2	3.6
Some college	25.7	33.9	28.1	9.5	2.8
Bachelor's degree or higher	38.5	35.6	19.8	4.7	1.5
Family income					
<$35000	26.1	26.5	29.8	12.8	4.7
$35000–$49999	31.8	31.9	26.3	8.0	2.0
$50000–$74999	36.0	32.6	23.9	6.2	1.4
$75000–$99999	40.4	34.0	20.7	4.1	0.8
$100000 or more	49.4	31.0	15.3	3.5	0.8
Health insurance coverage					
Under 65 years					
Private insurance	45.1	32.7	18.1	3.4	0.7
Medicaid	25.8	23.5	28.4	15.0	7.3
Other insurance	33.9	24.9	24.7	11.4	5.1
Uninsured	32.9	29.2	28.1	8.1	1.7
Over 65 years					
Medicare	13.1	26.2	34.9	19.3	6.6

Source: National Center for Health Statistics (2011). *Summary health statistics for the US Population: National Health Interview Survey, 2010.* Bethesda, MD: National Center for Health Statistics

Occupation, Industry, and Employment Status

Morbidity patterns related to the workforce can be examined in terms of occupation, industry, and employment status. Occupation refers to the type of job that a person performs in the economic system regardless of industry. Occupation can be examined in terms of occupational status (e.g., blue-collar, white-collar, professional) or in terms of specific occupations. Industry refers to the sector of the economy in which an occupation is located (e.g., manufacturing, retail trade, public administration). The same occupation (e.g., secretary) may be found in all industrial sectors.

There is a direct and positive relationship between the status of the occupation one holds and morbidity. In general, the higher the occupational prestige, the better the health status. Those at lower occupational levels tend to be characterized by higher rates of morbidity and disability. Like the poor and the uneducated, they tend to be characterized both by more conditions and by more serious conditions. Levels of disability (as measured by restricted activity days and lost days from work and school) are higher for lower occupational levels.

One of the few studies on morbidity and occupational status found that living and working conditions, psychosocial stress, and health and sickness behavior were more deleterious among blue-collar workers than among white-collar workers, resulting in higher morbidity and mortality rates for blue-collar workers. Psychosocial stressors at work were related to mental strain, perceived health, and absenteeism. Stress symptoms were strongly associated with perceived health, locomotor symptoms, smoking, drinking, and absenteeism. In follow-up research the baseline indicators of stress predicted future chronic illness and angina pectoris, but not hypertension or myocardial infarction. The study suggests that the psychosocial stress affecting blue-collar workers may be causally linked to such indicators of morbidity as perceived health, bodily symptoms, and sickness behavior (Aro and Hasan 1987). A more recent study (Sims et al. 2011) found that poorly educated people in low-status jobs had a higher prevalence of diabetes than highly educated people in management jobs.

Although attempts have been made to link mental disorder with occupational status, the results have been less clear-cut. Occupational status is a difficult concept to operationalize and is further complicated by American society's complex stratification system. It has been argued that an association exists between occupational status and mental health status in that the lower the former, the higher the latter. Such a monotonic relationship has not been convincingly demonstrated, however.

Mortality rates and longevity vary directly with occupational status. Mortality rates for professionals are significantly lower than those for unskilled laborers, for example. A study in Sweden and Germany found a link between mortality and occupational status, with the risk of death for the lowest occupational group (unskilled laborers) being nearly twice that of the highest (professionals), although the authors note that income and education are confounding factors (Geyer et al. 2006). Additional research by Rogers et al. (2000) has reaffirmed this finding as it relates to the US population. The causes of death for those lower in terms of occupational status are similar to those for the poor and uneducated.

The relationship between various occupations and industries and health status can also be examined. It is found that certain occupations tend to be characterized by inordinately high levels of both morbidity and mortality. High-morbidity occupations often include those whose workers are exposed to environmental risks. Healthcare workers, for example, are characterized by high levels of work-related injuries and illnesses (but very low levels of work-related deaths). The single most dangerous occupation today is cellphone tower workers, having recently edged out commercial fisherman and lumberjacks. Some professions such as psychiatry and dentistry are noteworthy for their high suicide rates.

It is also found that certain industries tend to be characterized by inordinately high levels of both morbidity and mortality. Among the standard industrial categories utilized by the US Department of Labor, the industry recording the highest level of occupational illnesses and injuries is manufacturing with a rate of 373 per 1000 workers in 2008. This compares to a rate of 10 per 1000 for utilities workers. The highest death rates by industry in 2008 were recorded by farming/fishing/forestry with 30.4 deaths per 100000 employed workers. This compares to finance and insurance with 0.3 deaths per 100000 workers (National Center for Health Statistics 2010a, b). While those employed in healthcare are characterized by a relatively high level of occupation-related illness and injury, the death rate for healthcare and social assistance workers is only 0.5 per 100000.

One other consideration when examining work-related morbidity is the issue of employment status. This issue may be more significant than that of occupational differentials and has garnered renewed attention in the light of current high levels of unemployment. When the employed are compared to the unemployed, clear-cut differences surface in terms of physical and mental illness (Brown et al. 2012). The unemployed appear to be sicker in terms of most health status indicators, with higher levels of morbidity and disability than the employed. While it could be argued that poor health leads to unemployment, it has been found that otherwise healthy individuals who have undergone loss of employment often develop symptoms of health problems. In fact, even perceived threats to job security have been associated with an increase in morbidity (Ferrie et al. 1998). It has also been suggested that, among those who cannot find employment, developing an illness serves as something of a rationale for a failure to find work. Recent research on 54 countries (including the US) found that the 2008 global recession contributed to a jump in suicide rates. The suicide rate in 2009 was 6.4 % higher than expected, with males aged 45–64 exhibiting the greatest risk of suicide during this period (Chang et al. 2013).

The same pattern holds for employment status and mental illness. The unemployed tend to be characterized by higher levels of mental illness symptoms than the employed. In fact, for both physical and mental disorders, it has been suggested that the lack of social integration resulting from unemployment serves as a "trigger" for various health problems. (See Exhibit 7.4 for a discussion of factors that might trigger the onset of disease.)

Not surprisingly, the disability level is lower for those in the labor force than for those not in the labor force. However, the American Community Survey found that 33.4 % of working-age individuals with a disability were employed.

Exhibit 7.4 "Triggers" for the Onset of Disease

In recent years there has been an increasing interest in the notion of "triggers" for the onset of disease. While the idea that many diseases lie dormant and only emerge in response to some trigger is not new, the scientific study of this phenomenon has only recently come to the fore. Speculation related to disease triggers goes back several decades in the US Antonovsky (1979) raised the question of, given the ubiquity of disease, why is it that some people get sick and others do not. Noting that most people carry diseases in their latent forms, he suggested the possibility of factors that trigger the onset of disease or, conversely, deter the onset of disease.

A variety of factors are thought to trigger the onset of disease, some of which are relatively tangible (e.g., air pollution) while others are more subjective (e.g., self-esteem). Environmental factors have certainly been cited as potential triggers. Nitrates may be an environmental trigger for Alzheimer's, diabetes, and Parkinson's disease. Environmental triggers for asthma and autism have been cited as well. Many cancers, along with a plethora of other diseases, are thought to emerge as a result of environmental triggers.

The presence of stress in the life of the individual has increasingly been cited as a factor in the onset of disease. Physical stress from a traumatic event or even something as routine as pregnancy may cause certain diseases to activate. Stress can contribute to a variety of physiological effects with the potential to trigger a defensive response to disease or actually promote disease. The stress response has implications for the cardiovascular, respiratory, muscular, metabolic, immune, and central nervous systems. As noted by Chrousos (1998), "the…effects of the stress response constitute biological pathways along which a person's experiences, living and working conditions, interpersonal relationships, lifestyle, diet, personality traits, and general socioeconomic status can affect the body."

Much of the discussion surrounding triggers to disease focuses on the impact of potential triggers on individuals, a situation of limited concern for demographers. At the same time, however, it could be argued that many of the suspected triggers actually affect groups of people, groups often identified in terms of their demographic attributes. Thus, not everyone in the population is at equal risk of exposure to environmental triggers; members of certain demographic groups face more dangers than those in other population subgroups. Further, the types of stress faced by members of certain groups may be more likely to trigger disease onset within vulnerable populations than the stress faced by members of groups that have adequate resources for coping with stressful events.

References

Antonovsky, A. (1979). *Health, stress, and coping*. San Francisco: Jossey-Bass.
Chrousos, G. P. (1998). Stressors, stress, and neuroendocrine integration of the adaptive response. *Annals of the New York Academy of Sciences, 851*, 311–335.

Religion

Perhaps the most poorly documented relationship of a demographic variable with morbidity is the link between religion and health status. Religion as it relates to morbidity in the US society has received limited attention compared to other demographic variables, and information linking religion affiliation or religiosity with morbidity is fragmented. However, a growing body of empirical evidence suggests that religious involvement has an impact on the level of morbidity (Oman et al. 2005).

Donahue and Benson (1995) found religious commitment to be associated with higher perceived well-being among adolescents. Studies also have associated higher frequency of church attendance with lower blood pressure and less physical disability (Oman et al. 2005). The lifestyles associated with strict religious groups such as Mormons and Seventh Day Adventists have been found to contribute to their higher health status. Some religion-specific differentials in morbidity that have been found are typically not in terms of overall prevalence, but in regard to group-specific conditions. For example, the Jewish population in the US is characterized by higher levels of some conditions and lower levels of others. However, it is usually argued that these differences reflect cultural variations rather than religious differences.

The findings on the association between religion and mental illness are not particularly clear-cut (Levin 2010). However, several studies have indicated that religion serves as something of a deterrent to the onset of psychiatric problems (Kendler et al. 2003). In a review of 93 studies conducted prior to 2000, two-thirds found lower rates of depression or fewer depressive symptoms among the more religious (Koenig et al. 2001). A review of studies conducted more recently found an association (albeit it weak) between religious involvement and depression (Smith, McCullough and Poll 2003). Further, among patients with serious medical conditions, the rate of depression has been found to be higher among those with no religious affiliation (Koenig 2007). Among those within this patient population who were depressed, those who participated in religious activities were able to eliminate depressive symptoms much faster.

Substance abuse may be viewed as either a physical or mental condition depending on the context. Koenig et al. (2001) found considerably less substance abuse among the more religious based on their review of previous studies; rates for substance use and substance abuse were found to be much higher for the non-religious than the religious in the subsequent national surveys (National Center on Addiction and Substance Abuse 2009).

Hummer et al. (1999) found a clear relationship between church attendance and mortality rates. People who never attend church services exhibit a risk of death 1.87 times than those who attend services two or more times per week. This calculates out to a 7-year difference in life expectancy (at age 20) between non-attenders and frequent attenders. Koenig et al.'s 2001 review of previous studies found that those who were deemed to be religious experienced fewer suicides than the non-religious.

Exhibit 7.5 presents the prevalence of various health conditions by selected population characteristics. Exhibit 7.6 describes the health risks exhibited by vulnerable populations. Exhibit 7.7 describes the situation with regard to health disparities in the U.S.

Exhibit 7.5 Age-Adjusted Prevalence of Selected Health Conditions for Adults by Selected Characteristics, US, 2010

Characteristic	Diabetes (%)	Kidney disease (%)	Arthritis (%)	Asthma (%)	Cancer (%)
Total	8.8	1.7	21.6	8.2	8.2
Age					
18–44 years	2.8	0.7	7.1	8.1	2.2
45–64 years	12.3	2.0	30.3	8.4	9.9
65–74 years	22.0	3.5	49.0	8.7	20.4
75 years and over	21.7	10.0	4.7	7.4	27.2
Sex					
Male	9.8	1.6	18.8	5.8	7.9
Female	8.0	1.7	24.1	10.3	8.6
Racial ethnicity					
White	8.2	1.6	21.8	8.0	8.8 %
Black	12.9	2.8	22.4	7.8	5.3
Asian	9.1	0.9	12.1	10.5	3.1
American Indian	16.3	1.1	25.5	10.5	11.0
Hispanic	13.2	2.1	15.6	6.9	2.7
Education					
Less than high school	14.7	3.1	24.6	7.7	7.1
High school diploma	10.6	1.8	26.4	7.2	8.6
Some college	10.3	2.2	27.7	9.6	10.7
Bachelor's degree or higher	7.1	1.0	20.2	10.6	10.4
Family income					
<$35000	11.2	2.7	24.6	9.9	7.9
$35000–$49999	9.4	1.9	21.6	8.1	8.6
$50000–$74999	9.0	1.2	22.6	7.6	8.0
$75000–$99999	40.4	34.0	20.7	6.9	9.2
$100000 or more	49.4	31.0	15.3	7.7	8.7
Health insurance coverage					
Under 65 years					
Private insurance	5.3	0.3	14.7	7.7	5.1
Medicaid	12.3	3.9	23.7	13.9	6.4
Other insurance	12.8	2.6	27.0	11.3	8.1
Uninsured	5.6	1.4	11.7	6.6	3.0
Over 65 years					
Medicare	13.1	26.2	34.9	7.2	21.6

Source: National Center for Health Statistics (2011). *Summary health statistics for the US Population: National Health Interview Survey, 2010.* Bethesda, MD: National Center for Health Statistics

Exhibit 7.6 Vulnerable Populations

Vulnerable populations (from a healthcare perspective) are those segments of the population that are at inordinate health risk due to their particular attributes. Vulnerable populations include the economically disadvantaged, racial and ethnic minorities, the uninsured, low-income children, the elderly, the homeless, those with human immunodeficiency virus (HIV), and those with other chronic health conditions, including severe mental illness. The vulnerable may also include rural residents, who often encounter barriers to accessing healthcare services. The vulnerability of people in these categories may be exacerbated by race, ethnicity, age, sex, and factors such as income, insurance coverage (or lack thereof), and absence of a usual source of care. Their health and healthcare problems intersect with social factors, including housing quality, poverty, and educational attainment.

Although each vulnerable subpopulation can be small in size, as a group these subpopulations represent a substantial number of persons who are at inordinate risk. Certain settings have high concentrations of at-risk populations, including nursing homes, correctional facilities, and homeless shelters. Infectious diseases that emerge from such settings or within these populations can eventually spread to the general population.

The health domains of vulnerable populations can be divided into three categories: physical, psychological, and social. Those with physical needs include high-risk mothers and infants, the chronically ill and disabled, and persons living with HIV/acquired immunodeficiency syndrome. In the psychological domain, vulnerable populations include those with chronic mental conditions, such as schizophrenia, bipolar disorder, major depression, and attention-deficit/hyperactivity disorder, as well as those with a history of alcohol and/or substance abuse. In the social realm, vulnerable populations include those living in abusive families, the homeless, immigrants, and refugees. The most vulnerable may be affected by more than one domain and have multiple problems, facing more significant comorbidities and cumulative risks of their illness.

The size of the vulnerable population is increasing, not only as the ranks of the uninsured have grown, but as the population ages. For instance, the number of individuals with chronic medical conditions has risen from 125 million in 2000 to 141 million in 2012, with an overall increase to 171 million people expected by 2030.

Shi and Stevens evaluated data on 32374 adults from the 2000 National Health Interview Survey and identified three risk factors for poor access to healthcare: low income, lack of health insurance, and lack of regular care. They found that those without insurance were seven times less likely to get the healthcare they need and 4.5 times less likely to not fill a prescription.

(continued)

Exhibit 7.6 (continued)

Meanwhile, adults with low incomes were more likely to delay or not receive necessary medical, dental, and mental healthcare and to not fill prescriptions. Overall, researchers found that about 1 of 5 US adults has multiple risk factors for unmet health needs, creating up to a fivefold difference in the rates of these unmet needs, such as delayed medical care between those with the greatest number of risk factors and those with the least.

Source: *American Journal of Managed Care* (2006). Vulnerable populations: Who are they? November 01, 2006 AJMC.com. Retrieved June 1, 2013, from http://www.ajmc.com/publications/supplement/2006/2006-11-vol12-n13suppl/nov06-2390ps348-s352/1

Exhibit 7.7 Health Disparities

Health disparities are, according to the National Institutes of Health, differences in the incidence, prevalence, mortality, and burden of diseases and other adverse health conditions that exist among specific population groups in the US. Much of this chapter has been devoted to the differences that exist in morbidity patterns between various subsets of the US population. "Differences" become "disparities" when they reflect disadvantages inherent in the status of affected parties and/or are the consequences of an inequitable and/or discriminatory system. Health disparities in the US exist along a number of different dimensions—based on income, on educational level, on marital status, on community type, and even by region of the country.

While many segments of the population—especially those considered to be "vulnerable" exhibit disparities, the groups most affected by disparities appear to be non-whites (particularly African-Americans) and the poor. We know that compared to whites, African-Americans have higher rates of many types of acute and chronic conditions, with the differences more profound for chronic problems. African-Americans are also considerably more likely to suffer from a disability. For many conditions, the same health problem is more severe for African-Americans than for whites and results in more negative outcomes.

The reasons for the existence of disparities in morbidity within the US population are numerous and complex. The very diversity of the population almost guarantees that different subgroups will have different characteristics. Even so, there are some factors that are noted for their contribution to disparities in morbidity. Certainly poverty is the most prominent of these and the attributes of a poverty-level existence that contribute to ill-health have been well documented, running the gamut from poor diets to inadequate housing to simply an unsafe, unhealthy daily existence. Woven into the overt effects of poverty is the underlying stress that results from fighting to survive on a daily basis.

(continued)

Exhibit 7.7 (continued)

Other factors that are associated with poor health include educational level, employment status and occupation (all of which are associated with income of course). Lifestyles also contribute to disparities in morbidity, with subgroups within society pursuing varying lifestyles that have consequences for their health status—either positive or negative. Noteworthy are those subgroups whose members are involved in unhealthy, risky, or otherwise health-negative behaviors.

The relationship between disparities in morbidity and various demographic attributes is complicated, and observed relationships often require considerable parsing to derive the true association. Sociologist David Williams (2005) reviewed several years' worth of health experiences for whites and African-Americans and examined a wide range of factors to determine their correlation with morbidity. He found, like most everyone else, a clear disparity in health status between whites and African-Americans. However, when he held income constant, *most* of the disparity between whites and African-Americans disappeared. However, there was still some residual disparity that could not be explained by socioeconomic differences.

That raises the question: How do we account for the fact that being African-American carries an increased health risk. Is it racism? A lifetime of being a second-class citizen? The persistent stress of day-to-day survival? This dimension of disparity-causing factors is only now being explored in depth, and a recent review of research by Williams and Mohammed (2009) has revealed a relationship between a lifetime of discrimination and its associated stress and poorer health status.

One final consideration relates to the contribution the healthcare system itself makes to disparities in disease and death. Phelan and Link (2005) suggest that our capacity to control disease and death in combination with existing social and economic inequalities create disparities based on race and socioeconomic status. While the ability of medical science to reduce disease and postpone death is generally seen as a positive benefit, the benefit is unequally distributed, thereby exacerbating existing disparities.

References

Cutts, T. (2011). The Memphis Congregational Health Network Model: Grounding ARHAP Theory. In J. R. Cochrane, B. Schmid, & T. Cutts (Eds.), *When religion and health align: mobilizing religious health assets for transformation* (pp. 193–206). Pietermaritzburg, South Africa: Cluster.

Phelan, J. C., & Link, B. J. (2005). Controlling disease and creating disparities: A fundamental cause perspective. *The Journals of Gerontology Series B* 60B (Special Issue II): 27–33.

Williams, D. R. (2005). The health of U.S. racial and ethnic populations. *Journal of Gerontology: Series B, 60B* (Special Issue II): 53–62.

Williams, D. R., Mohammed, S. A., Leavell, J., et al. (2010). Race, socioeconomic status, and health: Complexities, ongoing challenges, and research opportunities. *Annals of the New York Academy of Sciences, 1186*, 69–101.

References

American Journal of Managed Care. (2006). *Vulnerable populations: who are they?* November 01, 2006 AJMC.com. Retrieved June 1, 2013, from http://www.ajmc.com/publications/supplement/2006/2006-11-vol12-n13suppl/nov06-2390ps348-s352/1.

American Lung Association. (2011). *Trends in asthma morbidity and mortality.* Washington, DC: American Lung Association.

Antonovsky, A. (1979). *Health, stress and coping.* San Francisco, CA: Jossey-Bass.

Aro, S., & Hasan, J. (1987). Occupational class, psychosocial stress and morbidity. *Annals of Clinical Research, 19*(2), 62–68.

Aseltine, R. H., & Kessler, R. C. (1993). Marital disruption and depression in a community sample. *Journal of Health and Social Behavior, 34*(3), 237–251.

Australian Bureau of Statistics. (1997). *National survey of mental health and wellbeing.* Canberra, Australia: Australian Bureau of Statistics.

Brandon, L. J., & Proctor, L. (2010). Comparison of health perceptions and health status in African-Americans and Caucasians. *Journal of the National Medical Association, 102*(7), 590–597.

Brown, J., Demou, E., Tristram, M. A., et al. (2012). Employment status and health: Understanding the health of the economically inactive population in Scotland. *BMC Public Health, 12*, 327.

Chang, S.-S., Stuckler, D., Yip, P., et al. (2013). Impact of 2008 global economic crisis on suicide: Time trend study in 54 countries. *British Medical Journal, 347*, f5239.

Chrousos, G. P. (1998). Stressors, stress and neuroendocrine integration of the adaptive response. *Annals of the New York Academy of Sciences, 851*, 311–335.

Cutts, T. (2011). The Memphis congregational health network model: Grounding ARHAP theory. In J. R. Cochrane, B. Schmid, & T. Cutts (Eds.), *When religion and health align: Mobilizing religious health assets for transformation* (pp. 193–206). Pietermaritzburg, South Africa: Cluster Publications.

Donahue, M. J., & Benson, P. L. (1995). Religion and the well-being of adolescents. *Journal of Social Issues, 51*(2), 145–160.

Eaton, N. R., Krueger, R. F., Keyes, K. M., Hasin, D. S., Balsis, S., Skodol, A. E., et al. (2011). An invariant dimensional liability model of gender differences in mental disorder prevalence: Evidence from a national sample. *Journal of Abnormal Psychology.* Retrieved from http://www.apa.org/news/press/releases/2011/08/mental-illness.aspx.

Evans, G. W., & Kim, P. (2007). Childhood poverty and health: Cumulative risk exposure and stress dysregulation. *Psychological Science, 8*(11), 953–957.

Ferrie, J. E., Shipley, J. J., Marmot, M. G., Stansfeld, S. A., & Smith, G. D. (1998). An uncertain future: The health effects of threats to employment security in white-collar men and women. *American Journal of Public Health, 88*(7), 1030–1036.

Geyer, S., Hemstrom, O., Peter, R., et al. (2006). Education, income, and occupational class cannot be used interchangeably in social epidemiology. *Journal of Epidemiology and Community Health, 60*(9), 804–810.

Gijsbers van Wijk, C. M. T., & Kolk, A. M. (1997). Sex differences in physical symptoms: The contribution of symptom perception theory. *Social Science & Medicine, 45*(2), 231–246.

Hollingshead, A. B., & Redlich, F. C. (1958). *Social class and mental illness: A community study.* New York: Wiley.

Hoyert, L., & Xu, J. (2012). *Deaths: preliminary data from 2011.* Retrieved from http://www.cdc.gov/nchs/data/nvsr/nvsr61/nvsr61_06.pdf.

Hummer, R. A., Rogers, R. G., Nam, C. B., & Ellison, C. G. (1999). Religious involvement and US adult mortality. *Demography, 36*(May), 273–285.

Jitender, S., Afifi, T. O., McMillan, K. A., & Asmundson, G. J. G. (2011). Relationship between household income and mental disorders: Findings from a population-based longitudinal study. *Archives of General Psychiatry, 68*(4), 419–427.

Kendler, K. S., Liu, X.-Q., Gardner, C. O., et al. (2003). Dimensions of religiosity and their relationship to lifetime psychiatric and substance use disorders. *American Journal of Psychiatry, 160*(3), 496–503.

Kessler, R. C., Berglund, P., Demler, O., et al. (2003). The epidemiology of major depressive disorder: Results from the National Comorbidity Survey Replication (NCS-R). *Journal of the American Medical Association, 289*(23), 3095–3105.

Koenig, H. G. (2007). Religion and depression in older medical inpatients. *American Journal of Geriatric Psychiatry, 15*, 282–291.

Koenig, H. G., McCullough, M. L., & Larsen, D. B. (2001). *Handbook of religion and health*. New York: Oxford University Press.

Lantz, P. M., House, J. S., Lepkowski, J. M., et al. (1998). Socioeconomic factors, health behaviors, and mortality: Results from a nationally representative prospective study of US adults. *Journal of the American Medical Association, 279*(21), 1703–1708.

Levin, J. (2010). Religion and mental health: Theory and research. *International Journal of Applied Psychoanalytic Studies*. Retrieved from http://www.isreligion.org/wp-content/uploads/levin_religion_mental_health.pdf.

Lloyd-Jones, D., Adams, R. J., Brown, T. M., et al. (2010). Heart disease and stroke statistics—2010 update: A report from the American Heart Association. *Circulation, 121*, e1–e170.

Mathews, T. J., & MacDorman, M. F. (2013). Infant mortality statistics from the 2009 period linked birth/infant death data set. *National Vital Statistics Reports, 61*(8).

Maughan, B., Iervolino, A. C., & Collishaw, S. (2005). Time trends in child and adolescent mental disorders. *Current Opinion in Psychiatry, 18*(4), 381–385.

Mead, H., Cartright-Smith, L., Jones, K., et al. (2008). *Racial and ethnic disparities in U.S. health care: A chartbook*. Retrieved from http://www.commonwealthfund.org/Publications/Chartbooks/2008/Mar/Racial-and-Ethnic-Disparities-in-U-S--Health-Care--A-Chartbook.aspx.

Meyers, L. (2006). Asian-American mental health. *APA Monitor, 37*(2), 44.

Murali, V., & Oyebode, F. (2004). Poverty, social inequality and mental health. *Advances in Psychiatric Treatment, 10*, 216–224.

National Center for Health Statistics. (2010). *Death rates for 358 selected causes, by 10-year age groups, race, and sex: United States, 1999–2007*. Bethesda, MD: National Center for Health Statistics. Retrieved from http://www.cdc.gov/nchs/data/dvs/MortFinal2007_Worktable12.pdf.

National Center for Health Statistics. (2012). *Health, United States 2012*. Bethesda, MD: National Center for Health Statistics.

National Center on Addiction and Substance Abuse. (2009). *Spirituality and religion reduce risk of substance abuse*. Retrieved from http://www.casacolumbia.org/templates/PressReleases.asp x?articleid=115&zoneid=48.

Oman, D., Kurata, J. H., Strawbridge, W. J., & Cohen, R. D. (2005). Religious attendance and cause of death over 31 years. *International Journal of Psychiatry in Medicine, 32*(1), 69–89.

Phelan, J. C., & Link, B. J. (2005). Controlling disease and creating disparities: A fundamental cause perspective. *The Journals of Gerontology Series B, 60*(Special Issue II), 27–33.

Pleis, J. R., Ward, B. W., & Lucas, J. W. (2010). Summary health statistics for U.S. adults: National Health Interview Survey, 2009. *Vital Health Statistics 10, 249*, 1–207.

Riolo, S. A., Nguyen, T. A., Greden, J. F., & King, C. A. (2005). Prevalence of depression by race/ethnicity: Findings from the National Health and Nutrition Examination Survey III. *American Journal of Public Health, 95*(6), 998–1000.

Rogers, R. G., Hummer, R. A., & Nam, C. B. (2000). *Living and dying in the USA: Behavioral, health and social differentials of adult mortality*. New York: Academic.

Seeff, L. C., & McKenna, M. T. (2003). Cervical cancer mortality among foreign-born women living in the United States, 1985 to 1996. *Cancer Detection and Prevention, 27*(3), 203–208.

Shoenborn, C. A. (2004). Marital status and health: 1999–2002. *Advance Data* (No. 351). Hyattsville, MD: National Center for Health Statistics.

Sims, M., Diez-Roux, A. V., Boykin, S., et al. (2011a). The socioeconomic gradient of diabetes prevalence, awareness, treatment, and control among African Americans in the Jackson Heart Study. *Annals of Epidemiology, 21*, 892–898.

Sims, M., Diez-Roux, A. V., Dudley, A., et al. (2011b). Perceived discrimination and hypertension among African Americans in the Jackson Heart Study. *American Journal of Public Health, 102*(Suppl 2), S258–S265.

Smith, T.B., McCullough, M.E., and J. Poll (2003). Religiousness and Depression: Evidence for a Main Effecdt and the Moderating Influence of Stressful Life Events, *Psychological Bulletion 129*(4):614–636.

U.S. Department of Health and Human Services. (1999a). *Mental health: A report of the surgeon general—Executive summary.* Rockville, MD: U.S. Department of Health and Human Services, Substance Abuse and Mental Health Services Administration, Center for Mental Health Services, National Institutes of Health, National Institute of Mental Health.

U.S. Department of Health and Human Services. (1999b). *Mental health: Culture, race and ethnicity, supplement to mental health: A report of the surgeon general—Executive summary.* Rockville, MD: U.S. Department of Health and Human Services, Substance Abuse and Mental Health Services Administration, Center for Mental Health Services, National Institutes of Health, National Institute of Mental Health.

Verbrugge, L. M. (1979). Marital status and health. *Journal of Marriage and the Family, 41*(2), 267–285.

Williams, D. R. (2005). The health of U.S. racial and ethnic populations. *Journal of Gerontology: Series B, 60B*(Special Issue II), 53–62.

Williams, D. R., Mohammed, S. A., Leavell, J., et al. (2010). Race, socioeconomic status, and health: Complexities, ongoing challenges, and research opportunities. *Annals of the New York Academy of Sciences, 1186,* 69–101.

World Health Organization, (N.D.). *Gender and women's mental health.* Retrieved from http://www.who.int/mental_health/prevention/genderwomen/en/.

Xu, J., Kochanek, K. D., Murphy, S. L., & Tejada-Vera, B. (2010). Deaths: Final data for 2007. *National Vital Statistics Reports, 58,* 19 (May 20).

Additional Resources

Abraham, L. K. (1993). *Mama might be better off dead.* Chicago, IL: University of Chicago Press.

Idler, E. L. (2014). *Religion as a social determinant of public health.* Washington, DC: American Public Health Association.

Montague, T. (2006). The dangers of being poor and nonwhite. *Rachel's democracy and health news* #848. Retrieved from http://www.rachel.org/en/node/6405.

Wailoo, K. (2000). *Dying in the city of the blues: Sickle cell anemia and the politics of race and health.* Chapel Hill, NC: North Carolina University Press.

Chapter 8
Current Patterns and Trends in US Morbidity

Even a casual review of patterns of morbidity in the US suggests that today's disease patterns are quite different from those exhibited a century ago or even a couple of decades ago. While the nature of morbidity can be expected to change over time in every society—through natural processes if nothing else—the dynamic nature of US society almost guarantees an ever-changing morbidity profile. Observed changes in US morbidity patterns are primarily a consequence of changes in the causes of morbidity and in the sources of threats to health. The emerging pattern of disease reflects changes in the environment (both natural and manmade), demographic trends, modifications to the social structure, lifestyles, and even the genetic makeup of the population.

Pre-modern societies typically exhibited a stable level of overall morbidity with only minor variations over time in the absence of any mitigating factors. While members of pre-modern societies were essentially at the whim of nature when it came to controlling their morbidity fate, members of modern industrial societies have much more control over the direction morbidity takes. This is not to say that the health of Americans is not affected by external forces—it clearly is—but that our personal health is much more directly influenced by the social context and the behavior of members of society and much more affected by our lifestyle choices than in the past. While pre-modern populations were essentially innocent victims of their environment, the individual and collective actions of members of US society are effectively the cause of most of their health problems.

For each dimension of morbidity addressed below, the current morbidity rate is presented along with any notable subpopulation figures and qualifying factors. This is followed by a review of longitudinal trends in morbidity to the extent that the data allow. Observed changes in morbidity patterns will be analyzed to determine causative factors when possible.

© Springer New York 2016

R.K. Thomas, *In Sickness and In Health*, Applied Demography Series 6,

DOI 10.1007/978-1-4939-3423-2_8

Trends in Perceived Health Status

In examining the changing level of morbidity within the US population, the question of appropriate measures arises. Unfortunately, there is no easy way to measure the overall health of the population at any point in time, much less compare overall morbidity for different time periods. One approach to tracking changes in morbidity levels would involve the measurement of overall health status. The most consistent source of data on both subjectively and objectively measured health status is the various surveys conducted by the federal government. An admittedly subjective approach involves self-assessments by respondents in surveys conducted by various federal agencies. Respondents are typically asked to rate their own health, using the response categories of "poor," "fair," "good," "very good," and "excellent." Once such ratings have been obtained from a number of respondents, an assessment of the health status of the population can be performed.

Based on data collected by the National Center for Health Statistics, it is found that two-thirds of the US population consider themselves to be in good or excellent health, while less than 10 % consider themselves to be in poor or fair health. Longitudinal data indicate that self-reported health status for Americans has gradually declined over the past 15 years.[1] The proportion reporting very good or excellent health was an age-adjusted 68.5 % in 1997 period, dropping to 65.6 % in 2011. The proportion reporting only fair or poor health status increased from 9.2 to 9.8 % during the same period (National Center for Health Statistics 2013). While the youngest age cohort (under 18 years) reported little change (from 2.1 to 2.0 %), all other age cohorts except seniors (65 years and older) reported decreases in health status. In contrast, the proportion of seniors reporting only fair or poor health status decreased from 26.7 to 24.4 %, while seniors reporting very good or excellent health increased from 38.0 to 41.4 %. (Exhibit 8.1 presents trends in self-reported health status.)

Exhibit 8.1 Trends in Self-Reported Health Status: US Selected Years

Response	1997 (%)	2005 (%)	2008 (%)	2011 (%)
Very good/excellent	68.5	66.5	66.0	65.6
Poor/fair	9.2	9.2	9.5	9.8

Source: National Center for Health Statistics

---

[1] 1997 is the earliest year for which questions were asked comparable to those used today, although data from reasonably similar surveys are available for selected previous years.

Both males and females reported a decline in health status over this time period, as did all racial groups except African-Americans. African-Americans, although historically experiencing the greatest health disparities, reported a decrease from 15.8 to 14.9 % in the proportion with fair or poor health. Hispanics experienced a less marked decrease in health status than other racial and ethnic groups.

All income groups reported a decrease in health status between 1997 and 2010, with the near-poor reporting the greatest decrease. Residents in the Northeast region reported a slight improvement in health status, while those residing in the three other regions (Midwest, South, and West) reported significant declines.

Data from 1987 suggest that the decline in self-reported health status between 1997 and 2010 reflects a reversal of previous trends. That is, up until the 1990s, fragmented data suggests that self-reported health status steadily improved, only to be followed by a decline over the past two decades.

Trends in the Type of Health Conditions

One approach to assessing a population's morbidity status involves a review of the *types* of health conditions that affect that population. The dramatic change in the morbidity profile of the US population over the past 100 years has involved a major shift from a predominance of acute conditions to a predominance of chronic conditions. This "epidemiologic transition" has engendered significant changes in the health status of the population and a potential increase in the level of morbidity. The increase in the prevalence of chronic conditions suggests a proportionately higher disease rate for increasingly larger segments of the population due to the fact that once chronic conditions are contracted they do not go away. Unlike acute conditions, chronic conditions have a cumulative effect. (See Exhibit 8.2 for a discussion of the epidemiologic transition.)

The Decline of Acute Conditions

The acute conditions that contributed heavily to the morbidity profile in the past have become increasingly less important in contemporary US society. Acute conditions are the dominant type of health problem in traditional societies (e.g., hunting-and-gathering and agricultural societies) and in developing countries where virtually everyone faces the same health risks. Younger populations are also more likely to be characterized by acute conditions, with the incidence of such conditions declining with age. Limited public health facilities, impoverishment, and a young age structure all contribute to a predominance of acute conditions in less developed societies. Further, the short average life expectancy in traditional societies mitigates against the appearance of many chronic conditions—that is, few people live long enough to develop chronic conditions.

The declining relevance of acute conditions within the US population is attributed to several factors. The elimination if not eradication of common communicable diseases that preyed on previous generations (and are still common in less developed societies) reduced the burden of acute conditions. Changing patterns of disease etiology also have played a role, with the threat of biologic pathogens being reduced and the impact of lifestyles and the environment increasing. From a demographic perspective, the changing age structure has been a major factor, with an aging population accumulating chronic conditions over time, leaving a smaller younger population to generate acute conditions.

While it is clear that acute conditions have become increasingly less significant within the US population over time, there are no aggregate measures available for systematically tracking changes in overall incidence. In the past the National Center for Health Statistics generated an aggregate measure of acute conditions but that practice was discontinued in the 1990s and the data are not available for replicating those measures today. This leaves us with the option of tracking the incidence of specific health acute conditions over time.

One source of data on acute conditions is the notifiable disease tracking system operated by the Centers for Disease Control and Prevention. As described in Chap. 3, the CDC has tracked communicable diseases for decades, providing the data necessary for monitoring specific diseases over time. Unfortunately, most common acute conditions do not fall under the purview of the CDC since they are not considered "notifiable" conditions. This system, thus, does not track common respiratory diseases, gastrointestinal problems, and the transient symptoms that constitute the bulk of acute conditions. Nevertheless, there is some benefit in examining the trends in the conditions that the CDC does track.

Exhibit 8.2   The Epidemiologic Transition

During the twentieth century, the United States and most other developed countries experienced an "epidemiologic transition." The epidemiologic transition involved a shift from a predominance of acute conditions to a predominance of chronic conditions within their populations. This phenomenon was primarily a consequence of the demographic transition affecting these countries earlier in the century along with advances in society's ability to manage health problems. In the former case, the aging of the population resulted in a dramatic change in the types of health conditions affecting its members. In the latter, the introduction of public health measures and, to a lesser degree, advances in clinical medicine eliminated certain health conditions and inadvertently brought other conditions to the fore.

While acute conditions result from pathogens in the environment or accidents, chronic diseases are characterized by a much more complex etiology. While acute conditions affect a cross-section of the population sometimes

(continued)

Exhibit 8.2 (continued)

seemingly at random, chronic diseases are much more selective in their impact. In the twentieth century, emergent chronic diseases reflected the combined effects of heredity, environment, lifestyles, and even access to healthcare. From a demographic perspective, this meant that, for the first time, demographically related disparities in health status would become noteworthy.

Prior to the epidemiologic transition, the most common health conditions were respiratory conditions, gastrointestinal conditions, infectious and parasitic conditions, and injuries. Even today, in traditional societies and populations with a younger age structure cholera, malaria, skin diseases, nutritional deficiencies, and similar acute conditions remain common. In wake of the epidemiologic transition, populations in developed countries and those with older populations are more likely to be affected by heart disease, cancer, diabetes, arthritis, chronic respiratory diseases, and other chronic conditions. As a practical matter, most members of traditional societies did not live long enough to contract chronic conditions and, when they did contract them, these conditions could not be managed and early death likely ensued.

It was not until the epidemiologic transition was well underway that the focus in medical science began to shift from acute conditions to chronic conditions. This shift has been a difficult transition for the US healthcare system due to the complexity of chronic disease etiology, its unpredictable progression, and its management challenges. More attention is now being paid to disease etiology (and, subsequently, disease prevention), disease progression and management and, importantly, the demographic disparities associated with chronic disease. For demographers and others concerned about the population's morbidity profile, the shift from a predominance of acute conditions to a predominance of chronic conditions has been momentous.

There has been considerable fluctuation in the number of cases of various communicable diseases over the past 40 years. While there were approximately 47000 reported cases of measles in 1970, for example, there were only 55 in 2012. This same downward trend can be seen over the same time period for mumps (105000 to 229 cases) and hepatitis A (56797 to 1562 cases). Some diseases, particularly sexually transmitted infections, reported a steady decline for decades only to experience a resurgence in recent years (Adams et al. 2014). On the other hand, the prevalence of AIDS steadily increased for several years, only to exhibit a sharp decline in the twenty-first century. (Data for selected notifiable diseases for five time periods are shown in Exhibit 8.3.)

Although the effect of the epidemiological transition has been to replace acute conditions with chronic conditions as the predominant health problems, we see that certain acute conditions continue to be reported at high rates and some, in fact, at rates that are unprecedented in the modern age. These include increased rates for a variety of acute conditions—including Legionnaire's disease, syphilis, pertussis,

Exhibit 8.3 Reported Cases of Selected Communicable Diseases in the US Selected Years

Disease	1970	1985	1996	2006	2012
AIDS	NA	8249	65475	36442	35631
Hepatitis A	56800	23200	49024	2579	1562
Hepatitis B	8300	26600	9994	4713	2895
Malaria	3051	1049	1542	1524	1503
Syphilis	91000	68000	11110	26598	49903
Gonorrhea	600000	911000	308737	356266	334836
Tuberculosis	37100	22200	19096	13754	9945
Measles	47400	2800	295	66	55
Mumps	105000	3000	658	314	229
Pertussis (whooping cough)	4200	3600	6467	15632	48277

Source: Centers for Disease Control and Prevention.

and valley fever (Adams et al. 2014). Many conditions that are associated with less healthy populations continue to generate a disturbing number of cases annually (e.g., tuberculosis, chicken pox, and salmonella). In addition, sexually transmitted infections remain at epidemic levels. While chronic conditions comprise the preponderance of health problems, the persistence exhibited by a number of acute conditions is noteworthy.

The Rise of Chronic Conditions

During the twentieth century chronic conditions displaced acute conditions as the predominant health problems and the leading causes of death. Common chronic conditions include arthritis, cardiovascular disease, cancer, diabetes, chronic pulmonary disease, and obesity. Chronic conditions are more common in industrialized societies and in those with an older age structure where they are referred to as "diseases of civilization." Conditions like heart disease, cancer, and diabetes were relatively uncommon among previous generations of Americans and remain rare among the populations of less developed societies today. (See Exhibit 8.4 for an overview of the diseases of civilization.)

Exhibit 8.4 "Diseases of Civilization"

A number of syndromes have been identified that were rare in traditional societies but have come to dominate the populations of modern, industrial societies. These conditions are collectively referred to as "diseases of civilization."

Overweight and Obesity

By themselves, overweight and obesity are not technically diseases, but they increase the risk of hypertension, type 2 diabetes, coronary heart disease (CHD), high cholesterol, stroke, gall bladder disease, some cancers (endometrial, breast, colon), sleep apnea, osteoarthritis, and Alzheimer's disease. In many people, obesity is also associated with increased levels of markers for inflammation and oxidative stress. For these reasons, trends in these conditions are highly relevant to disease patterns in human populations.

Childhood Overweight and Obesity

Overweight is also a serious health concern for children and adolescents. Data from two NHANES surveys (1976–1980 and 2003–2004) show that the prevalence of overweight is increasing: for children aged 2–5 years, the prevalence rate increased from 5.0 to 13.9 %; for those aged 6–11 years, the prevalence rate increased from 6.5 to 18.8 %; and for those aged 12–19 years, the prevalence rate increased from 5.0 to 17.4 %. *Healthy People 2010* identified overweight and obesity combined as one of ten leading health indicators and called for a reduction in the proportion of children and adolescents who are overweight or obese.

Diabetes

Diabetes has become more prevalent in all age groups in the US in the past 25 years. The best available evidence suggests that childhood type 1 diabetes showed a stable and relatively low prevalence over the first half of the twentieth century, followed by a clear increase that began at some time around or soon after the middle of the century, with an incidence now of three or four in a thousand. In recent years, type 2 diabetes, previously a phenomenon of later life and frequently associated with obesity, has become a significant and growing problem even among children.

Cardiovascular Disease

A sharp upturn in the prevalence of cardiovascular disease during the middle of the twentieth century led to considerable research into its origins and the means to prevent it. The recorded decline in death from cardiovascular disease during the past 25 years are due to a combination of factors including early detection, smoking reduction, blood pressure control, decrease in blood

(continued)

Exhibit 8.4 (continued)

cholesterol levels through dietary changes, and improvements in medical care, including emergency management and pharmaceutical interventions. Heart disease, however, remains the leading cause of death for both men and women in the US.

Hypertension

The prevalence of hypertension, defined as elevated blood pressure, has steadily increased in recent years. While genetics plays some part in the etiology of heart disease, lifestyles represent a greater influence today. Although data gaps make it difficult to determine changes in prevalence over many decades, evidence is sufficient to conclude that age-adjusted hypertension increased in the US population during the years 1988–2000.

Chronic conditions are also more prevalent in older populations as the acute conditions common to younger populations are supplanted by conditions that reflect lifestyles, health behaviors and the accumulative effect of a life of stress and wear and tear. In populations where chronic conditions are dominant a significant portion of the population is likely to be affected since, unlike acute conditions, chronic conditions do not resolve themselves.

Chronic conditions are the leading cause of illness, disability, and death in the United States. Today, chronic disease accounts for an estimated 80 % of contemporary health conditions. As of 2012, half of all adults (117 million) suffered from one or more chronic diseases; approximately 25 % reported two or more chronic conditions (Ward et al. 2014). These figures represent an increase over the 2001 level. The proportion of individuals exhibiting one or more chronic diseases increases with age, with 85 % for those 65 and over affected compared to 63 % for those 45–64 and 26 % for those 18–44. Based on NCHS studies, it has been found that the number of persons with one or more chronic diseases has increased from 16.1 % of the population (1999–2000 average) to 21.0 % (2009–2010 average). For males 45–64 the figure increased from 15.2 to 20.5 % and for females of the same age from 16.9 to 21.8 %. For those over 65 years, the increase in the proportion with one or more chronic diseases was from 37.2 to 45.9 %. These increases have been noted for both males and females and for all racial and ethnic groups.

One way in which to assess whether observed increases in chronic morbidity are real or simply reflect the growth of the elderly population is to compare rates for the same age cohort at different periods of time. Recent studies based on NCHS data have found an increase in the prevalence of chronic conditions (2 or more diseases) among those 45–64 from 16.1 to 21.0 % between 1999/2000 and 2009/2010 (Freid et al. 2012). These increases held for whites, blacks and Hispanics and all income groups. Another government analysis found for adults 45–64 years a significant increase between 2001 and 2010 in the proportions reporting 2–3 chronic diseases or 4 or more chronic diseases. For adults 65 years or older significant increases were also reported in the proportions reporting 2–3 chronic diseases or 4 or more chronic diseases (National Center for Health Statistics 2013). What is telling is the fact that contemporary cohorts report higher aggregate rates of chronic disease than comparable cohorts a generation ago.

In the past it was easy to rationalize increases in prevalence rates for chronic diseases. As the epidemiological transition unfolds, it is argued, the acute conditions characteristic of pre-modern populations are supplanted by the diseases of civilization characterizing modern populations. One should *expect* an increase in the prevalence of chronic conditions as the incidence of acute conditions declines. The available statistics, however, suggest that the prevalence of chronic disease is increasing at a faster rate than that warranted by demographic change. According to Crimmins and Beltran-Sanchez (2011), the prevalence of disease has actually increased more than would be anticipated simply based on the aging of the population.

Exhibit 8.5 Higher Disease Prevalence…or Better Diagnostics?

Any examination of changes in the level of morbidity raises the question of whether observed increases are a function of increased prevalence of disease or a function of improved diagnostics and/or better reporting. While there are suspicions that some of the reported increases in prevalence are a result of more cases being identified rather than a higher level of morbidity, there is no easy way to verify this. There is no aggregate measure that could be used that would provide an overall assessment of the extent to which better diagnostics or reporting results in an apparent higher morbidity rate.

Most would argue that whether observed increases in prevalence represent better diagnostics or not depends on the condition. The availability of improved diagnostic methods and thus more accurate and, often, earlier diagnoses varies from condition to condition. For conditions like breast and prostate cancer, improved diagnostics has resulted in an increase in the observed prevalence. However, death rates for these two cancers have not changed much, suggesting that the true prevalence rate has not changed and that more cases are being identified at earlier stages.

For other conditions (e.g., end-stage renal disease), an increase in prevalence has been observed in the absence of any changes in diagnostic capabilities, suggesting that the increase is, in fact, real.

The ability to answer this question is complicated by a couple of other factors. One of these is the dynamic nature of the criteria for the determination of a diagnosis. In the case of hypertension, for example, the threshold for high blood pressure has changed over time, making it difficult to compare observed prevalence from one time period to another. In other cases, the actual definition

(continued)

Exhibit 8.5 (continued)

for a condition may change over time making comparisons a challenge. In still other cases, a newly "discovered" condition (e.g., AIDS, Legionnaire's disease) may appear to experience a rapid increase that can be partly explained by the medical community's lag in recognizing the condition and, perhaps, not due to an actual increase.

One other complicating factor is that the (over) use of imaging technology may be contributing not only to better and earlier diagnoses but also to over-diagnosis. Markers that may not have been detected in the past are now readily revealed, often resulting in additional expensive and life-threatening tests to ascertain the nature of the condition. Critics argue that advanced diagnostic capabilities are being overutilized, resulting in false positives that could lead to unnecessary tests, surgery and other treatments (Bailey 2014).

Clearly, more research is required to determine the extent to which observed increases in chronic morbidity are a result of better diagnostics or actual increases in morbidity. This will remain a challenge for epidemiologists for years to come.

Reference

Bailey, J. (2014). *The end of healing*. Memphis, TN: The Healthy City Press.

Further, heart disease prevalence increased for both men and women over 65 years over the past two decades, with an increase of from 57.3 % (1988–1994 average) to 64.8 % (2003–2006 average) for males and from 64.5 to 75.3 % for females. The increase was similar for white males (from 56.0 to 64.1 %) and black males (from 70.5 to 79.9 %), for white females (from 63.7 to 74.0 %) and black females (from 74.7 to 86.9 %).

The prevalence of diagnosed diabetes increased in all US states, the District of Columbia, and Puerto Rico between 1995 and 2010, according to a study from the Centers for Disease Control and Prevention. During that time, the prevalence of diagnosed diabetes increased by 50 % or more in 42 states, and by 100 % or more in 18 states. Boyle (2010) predicts that one-third of the US population will suffer from diabetes by 2050. While all demographic subgroups have been affected, some have experienced greater increases than others. For example, diabetes prevalence is increasing among older men and women. The increase in diabetes prevalence has been even more dramatic for older African-American men, with rates for this group rising three times faster than those for white males.

The prevalence rate for stroke increased significantly for the US population over the past two decades. The rate per 1000 population increased from 9.8 in 1990 to 15.7 in 2010 (Feigin et al. 2014). Younger Americans are increasingly affected by stroke, with obesity, diabetes, and high blood pressure all contributing to an increase in the number of strokes reported. The prevalence rate for stroke increased by a quarter during this period for those 20–64.

Much of the increase in chronic morbidity has been attributed to the rise in obesity within the US population. The current prevalence of adult obesity (>35 %) reflects a rise from less than 15 % in the 1960s to 35 % by 2000. For children (6–11 years) the increase has been more dramatic, from 5 % in 1980 to 16 % in 2008. These increases have been observed essentially across all demographic groups. The prevalence of persons who are overweight and obese, characteristics that have been associated with increased prevalence of type 2 diabetes, hypertension, arthritis, and some cancers, has in effect more than doubled during the last 40 years.

Of particular concern for many is the apparent decline in the health status of US children. This phenomenon is described in Exhibit 8.6.

Exhibit 8.6 The Changing Health Status of American Children

The changing health status of American children has gained increasing attention among epidemiologists, public health officials, and policy makers in recent years. Although there appear to be a number of apparent trends, the tracking of childhood morbidity is often hindered by a lack of comparable historical data. It is clear that the risk of infant and childhood death—the major killer of children up through the middle of the twentieth century—has been mostly eliminated. This development reflects the introduction of medical, social, and public health measures that led to the elimination of the major infectious diseases and a subsequent reduction in infant and childhood mortality. (It should be noted, however, that the level of infant mortality exhibited by the US population is higher than that of comparable developed nations.)

What is less clear is the extent to which the current cohort of American children is more healthy or less healthy than previous cohorts. From the beginning of the twentieth century to the end of that century, the available data indicate a decline in childhood diseases such as measles and mumps by mid-century and a subsequent decline in chicken pox late in the twentieth century. At the same time, these data indicate an increase in most other acute and chronic conditions over the course of that century. The available data, in fact, suggests sharp increases in the prevalence of most childhood physical and mental health problems. Further, there appears to be an unprecedented increase in chronic health conditions.

Major increases are identified in the incidence or prevalence of asthma, other respiratory illnesses, allergies, and depression. Less dramatic but still important increases were noted for speech impediments, heart trouble, headaches/migraines, stomach problems, diabetes, epilepsy, and hypertension. In another study, asthma among children was found to increase from 3.6 % in 1980 to 9.7 % in 2007. There is growing evidence since then that American

(continued)

Exhibit 8.6 (continued)

children are experiencing increasing levels of diabetes and hypertension, chronic conditions typically associated with older adults. Data from other sources have verified increases in levels of obesity and asthma among physical illnesses and autism and ADHD among mental disorders. The National Longitudinal Survey of Youth (ages 2–8) found the prevalence of any chronic health condition to increase from 12.8 % in 1988 to 25.1 % in 2000 and then again to 26.6 % in 2006.

Over the last few decades, the rise in the rates of potentially disabling childhood conditions deserves special consideration. As early as the 1970s, when the rates of severe limitations grew from 2.7 to 3.7 %, Newacheck et al. (1984) found increasing rates of several health conditions, especially mental health conditions, asthma, orthopedic conditions, and hearing loss. Unfortunately, changes in the questions as part of the redesign of the National Health Interview Survey in 1997 prevent comparisons over the entire time period.

A study by the Institute of Medicine has described the increasing prevalence of childhood obesity as a "startling setback" for child health (Institute of Medicine 2006). Obesity is a risk factor for a number of serious health conditions, such as diabetes, that are, in turn, risk factors for disabilities. Based in part on concerns about the stigmatization of children and in part on concerns about the reliability of the body mass index (BMI) as a measure of fatness for children, CDC has used the term "overweight" for children who would be classified as overweight or obese on the basis of BMI criteria (Nihiser et al. 2004). An earlier IOM committee had concluded that the term "obesity" was appropriate for children 2 years of age and older who have a BMI at or above the 95th percentile for their age and sex groups. Exhibit 8.3 illustrates trends in childhood obesity.

There are major considerations with regard to interpreting these figures on childhood health status. Data from earlier historical periods are rare and typically not in a format that supports rigorous statistical analysis. Further, changes in the methods of reporting health conditions and, indeed, in the definitions of some conditions are mitigating factors. Clearly, methods of detection are much improved today, and the healthcare system is much more aggressive in ferreting out health conditions of various types. Nevertheless, the data that are available suggest that the health status of American children is not improving and, in fact, may be declining. Additional research is clearly required to confirm the trends that are suggested by available data.

Sources: Delaney L, and J P Smith (2012). Childhood Health: Trends and Consequences Over the Life Course, *The Future of Children*, *22*(1): 43–63.

Trends in Mental Illness Morbidity

While acquiring accurate data on psychiatric morbidity is more challenging than it is for physical illness, data collected through various sample surveys provide insights into the prevalence of psychiatric disorders in America. Since much of the psychiatric morbidity is undiagnosed, tallies of recorded cases, even if available, would not provide the complete picture of what some would consider an epidemic. Even the best-worded survey items may not elicit accurate and/or complete information on this phenomenon, and there is every reason to believe that the level of mental and emotional disorders characterizing the US population is higher than the estimates derived from sample surveys. Any analysis of psychiatric morbidity is further complicated by trends in the diagnosis of mental disorders exhibited by therapists (Nauert 2010).

By virtually any standard mental illness is widespread within the US population today. When the overall level of mental disorder is estimated, it is found that 1 in 17 Americans is characterized by a serious debilitating mental disorder (Kessler et al. 2005). In any given year, an estimated 26 % of the population suffers from an identifiable mental disorder, with 5.8 % of these being considered severe. The estimated lifetime occurrence of a serious mental disorder is 46 %, or nearly half of the population.

Based on surveys by the National Center for Health Statistics from the 1980s and 1990s up through 2011 it is possible to identify some trends in mental illness (National Center for Health Statistics 2013). Unfortunately, comparable data are not available for earlier periods (and most only from the mid-1990s), making the time-frame for trend analysis shorter than one would like. For adults, the proportion of the population reporting serious psychological distress was an age-adjusted 3.3 % for the 2010–2011 period. While this figure is little different from the 3.2 % recorded for the 1997–1998 timeframe, it does represent a meaningful increase over the lower rates recorded in the interceding years (e.g., 2.6 % for 1999–2000, 2.9 % for 2007–2008). The utilization of any type of mental health service increased from 13.0 to 14.6 % between 2002 and 2013. Interestingly, most of the increase in reported psychological distress could be attributed to the white population, with the rates for other racial and ethnic groups declining.

In terms of age, older adults were responsible for most of the increase, younger adults held steady, and seniors actually reported a decline in serious psychological distress over this 15-year period. Youth (age 12–17) reported an increase in major depressive episodes over the past year from 7.9 to 10.7 % between 2006 and 2013. While males consistently reported lower levels of psychological distress than females, the former accounted for more of the increase in reported levels. Young females (12–17) reported an increase in major depressive episodes from 13.1 to 16.2 %, compared to an increase from 5.0 to 5.3 % for males 12–17 years. Between 2006 and 2013, the proportion reporting severe psychiatric impairment increased from 5.5 to 7.7 %. The figures for females were 8.4 % and 12.0 % and for males 2.6 and 3.5 %. On the other hand, other NCHS studies found that the proportion of adults reporting severe psychiatric distress remained essentially the same between 1997/1998 and 2011–2012 (3.2 % and 3.1 %, respectively). The rate for African-Americans actually decreased during this time period.

Another study (Pal 2011) based on an analysis of national data from the Behavioral Risk Factor Surveillance System (BRFSS) found that in 2007 40 % of the population reported serious psychological distress. Rates were higher for women, the unmarried, and those living in poverty. Depression was the most common form of mental disorder, affecting 26 % of the population over a year's time (with 5.4 % affected in any 2-week time period). The survey's quality of life data indicated that for the 2004–2008 period US adults experienced on the average 3.4 mentally unhealthy days, and an astounding 10 % of adults experienced 14 or more mentally unhealthy days during the previous 30-day period. In examining trends in disability resulting from a mental disorder, Mojtabai (2011) found an increase in such disability from 2.0 % of the non-elderly population in 1997–1999 to 2.7 % in 2007–2009. Although some of the statistics presented below suggest an increase in psychiatric morbidity, data from the National Survey on Drug Use and Health (NSDUH) found a decline in the rate of depression among adults from 7.9 % in 2004 to 6.5 % in 2009 (Hedden et al. 2012).

Exhibit 8.7 How Crazy Are We? Case Finding in Mental Illness

Conventional wisdom suggests that as America became more industrialized and urbanized, the population also became crazier. Three or four generations ago, most citizens could live their entire lives without knowing anyone who was considered insane. There was the occasional "retard," "eccentric," or "truly certifiable" lunatic, of course, but for all practical purposes the American population was relatively free of the mentally ill.

Today, in stark contrast, it seems that mental illness is rampant. Startling figures are quoted for the number of individuals with various mental conditions, and millions of Americans are reported to be seeking treatment for some psychiatric condition. If "new" mental disorders (such as drug and alcohol abuse and eating disorders) are included, the size of the affected population is truly staggering. Unlike our forefathers, virtually everyone today knows someone who has been diagnosed and/or treated for one psychiatric condition or another.

What is the explanation for the apparent dramatic increase in the prevalence of mental disorders? Are we truly crazier as a people, or is there some other explanation? The answer to these questions depends on an understanding of case finding, or the manner in which individuals are identified as having a disorder or being a "case." Historically, a major problem has been a lack of data on the existence of mental illness within the population. No comprehensive

(continued)

Exhibit 8.7 (continued)

system for tracking mental disorders, or any condition for that matter, has ever been available. The fact that most mentally disturbed individuals in the past were handled informally—that is, by the family—meant that most never came to be officially recognized.

Until well into the twentieth century, the only source of information on the extent of mental disorders in the population was the official records of institutions charged with treating these cases. The main sources of such data were the asylums and mental institutions, along with other agencies of social control, such as jails, that for administrative purposes maintained records on their inmates. These records were thus utilized to develop estimates of the amount of mental disorder within the population.

Not surprisingly, such records indicated a strikingly low level of disorders within the US population, although those that were insane were *seriously* impaired. It was further determined from these records that most mentally ill individuals were nonwhite, poor, poorly educated, and/or of foreign descent.

Many of the deficiencies of this method of case finding were addressed with the introduction of the community survey method for identifying the prevalence of mental disorders. The nation's first known attempt at a community mental health study was conducted in 1917, and since then scores of community surveys have sought to determine the extent of mental illness within the US population. While there is little agreement as to which of the various studies most accurately reflects the true prevalence of mental disorder, all of the community surveys have had one thing in common: They have demonstrated that the prevalence of mental disorders identified using the reported-cases approach represents only the tip of the iceberg.

Then, how crazy are we *really*? After the administration of scores of community surveys, there is still little consensus. A review of 60 community studies conducted in the United States over several decades found estimates of prevalence ranging from less than 1 % to well over 50 % (Dohrenwend and Dohrenwend 1974). These studies included one rural area where the prevalence rate of functional psychiatric disorders was placed at 69 %! Another study, focusing on midtown Manhattan in New York City, found that less than one-fifth of the population was "well," about three-fifths exhibited mild forms of mental disorder, and one-fifth was characterized by severe psychiatric disorder. Later studies employing more sophisticated research methodologies have demonstrated less variation in the levels of disorder identified. A 1980 review of prevalence studies (Dohrenwend et al. 1980) found for all types of psychopathology that an average of 21 % of the population was affected. Applying statistically acceptable standards of preciseness, the review concluded that between 16 and 25 % of the US population has a clinically significant disorder at any point in time.

(continued)

Exhibit 8.7 (continued)

How is it possible to explain the apparent increase in mental disorders during this century, or the discrepancy between various studies conducted in presumably the same manner? These questions get at the heart of case finding. It is always the situation, and it is particularly true for mental illness, that what constitutes a "case" is what health professionals call a case. As the mental health field has evolved in US society, it has developed a much more precise classification system for mental disorders. One implication of this is a greater sensitivity to many conditions that, in the past, may have been passed off as eccentricities. In addition, over time, mental health officials have expanded their notion as to what constitutes a mental disorder. Many conditions that would have been considered historically as weirdness, immorality, or crime are now classified as psychiatric disorders. In the final analysis, there is probably no "true" prevalence of mental illness. Our level of sanity or insanity will always be a function of the case-finding techniques in use at the time and the public's notion of what constitutes mental illness.

References

Dohrenwend, B. P., & Dohrenwend, B. S. (1974). Social and cultural influences on psychopathology. *Annual Review of Psychology, 25*:417–47.
Dohrenwend, B. P., et al. (1980). *Mental illness in the United States: Epidemiological estimates*. New York: Praeger.

Trends in Disability

The amount of disability is another measure of the level of morbidity in the population and one that is exceptionally hard to specify. Even today there is little agreement as to the metrics that should be used of measure disability, and the approaches used have varied over time. Attempts at determining the absolute level of disability based on observed physical or mental defects have given way to one that conceptualizes disability in terms of functional capabilities.

Using criteria from the National Center for Health Statistics, the overall rate of all types of disability (for adults) in the US in 2010 was 28.7 %. Other metrics from NCHS indicate that for those 18 years and over 15.1 % of the population reported some limitation in basic activities. This figure was little changed from the 15.6 % recorded in 1997. Although the overall rate was little changed, the number of disabled in the population increased during this period from 60.9 million to 73.5 million. While the disability rate using this measure increased from 11.2 to 12.5 % for those 18–64 years, it actually decreased from 35.1 to 31.1 % for those 65 years and over. For Americans over 65 years, 5.2 % of men and 7.4 % of women needed help with activities of daily living. These figures increased with age with 2.6 % of men and 4.0 % of women 65–74 needing health with such activities compared to 14.9 % and 21.7 %, respectively, for those 85 and over (National Center for Health Statistics 2012).

These figures and others reinforce the notion that today's elderly are healthier (at least on some measures) than the "frail elderly" of past generations. A study sponsored by the American Hospital Association (MEDTAP 2004) found an overall decline in disability among seniors (i.e., 65 and over) from 26.2 % in 1980 to 19.7 % in 2000. When all forms of disability are considered (including institutionalization), it is found that the proportion of seniors who suffer from some kind of disability showed a steady decline between 1984 and 1999 from 25 to 20 % (Federal Interagency Forum on Aging-Related Statistics 2004). On the other hand, based on data from the National Center for Health Statistics, the proportion of the US population reporting activity limitation increased from 27.0 to 28.7 % from 1997 to 2010.

Data from the American Community Survey for 2013 (U.S. Census Bureau 2015) indicate a national disability rate of 12.6 % based on the criteria utilized for the ACS. This represents a slight increase from the 12.1 % recorded in 2008, the first year for which ACS data on disability are available. The rate recorded for males in 2013 was 12.4 % and for females 12.7 %. Native Americans reported the highest disability rate (17.0 %) with higher rates for whites (13.0 %) and African-Americans (13.9 %). Lower rates were recorded for Hispanics (8.7 %) and Asian-Americans (6.9 %). Disability rates tended to be inversely related to educational level, with those with a high school diploma or less recording 14.0 % compared to 8.2 % for those with a bachelor's degree or higher.

The BRFSS administered by the CDC measures disability based on self-reports of activity limitations.[2] The 2008 survey found that the rate of disability increased with age, with 13.4 % of those 18–44 reporting a disability, 27.4 % of those 45–64, and 37.8 % of those 65 and over (Armour 2010). The reported rate for females was 22.4 % compared to 21.1 % for males. The reported rate for whites and blacks was the same at 22.7 %, with Hispanics and Hawaiian/Pacific Islanders reporting lower rates and Asian-Americans reporting rates half that of whites and blacks (10.4 %). American Indians reported by far the highest rates (31.3 %). There was an inverse relationship between income and the prevalence of disability in the BRFSS survey, with those in the lowest income group ($15000 or less) reporting a rate of 38.8 % compared to 16.2 % for the highest income group ($50000+).

The 2008 BRFSS found that the rate of disability varies significantly from state to state (as illustrated in Exhibited 8.8). The highest rates were generally found in the South region and in the northwestern states. The lowest rates were generally found in the Midwest region. The 2013 ACS confirmed higher rates for the southern states but not for the northwestern states.

---

[2] Research should be noted that suggests the BRFSS survey may understate the level of disability within the population (Hall et al. 2012).

Exhibit 8.8

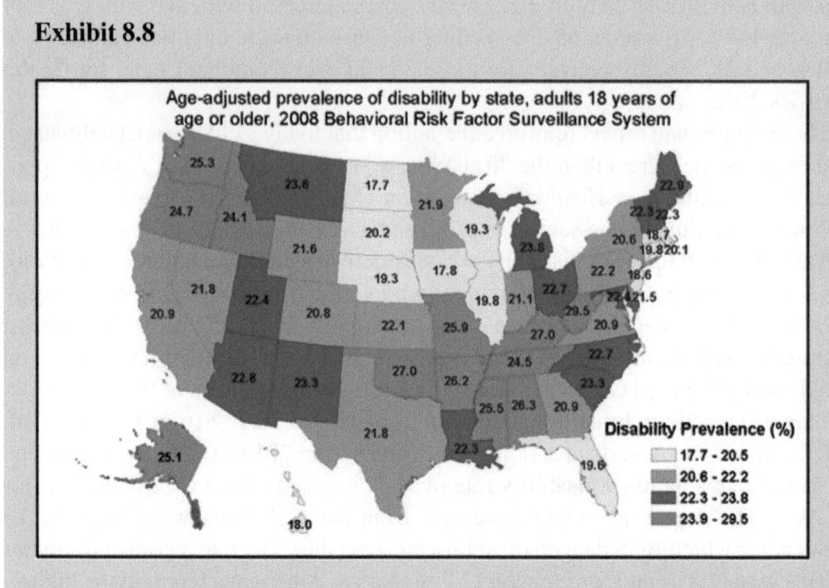

Age-adjusted prevalence of disability by state, adults 18 years of age or older, 2008 Behavioral Risk Factor Surveillance System

Source: Centers for Disease Control and Prevention, 2008 BRFSS survey.

One method of determining trends in disability is to track the number of disability claims approved by the Social Security Administration. Admittedly, the criteria for approval change over time making it difficult to draw definitive conclusions. However, based on an analysis of approved claims for disability it can be argued that the trend for awards per 1000 population for men, after a slight increase between 1985 and 1995, was more or less flat from 1985 to 2013 (Morrisey 2015). This trend essentially tracked the path that would have been predicted based on demographic change. The rate of claims per 1000 for women, however, increased during this period from 4 per 1000 insured persons to around 6 per 1000. The observed increase in the disability rate for women was thought to reflect demographic changes and the increased participation of women in the workforce rather than an actual increase in the disability level.

One condition potentially contributing to high rate of disability is preterm birth. For a variety of reasons, including the increased rates of survival of high-risk infants and the growth in the number of multiple births associated with certain fertility treatments, the numbers of infants born prematurely and with low birth weights have increased (Institute of Medicine 2006). For example, the rate of premature births (as a percentage of all births) increased from 10.6 % in 1990 to 12.5 % in 2004. Prematurity (birth before 37 weeks of completed gestation) and low birth weight (birth weight less than 2500 g) are risk factors for a number of short-term and long-term neurodevelopmental and other health problems and disabilities such as cerebral palsy, mental retardation, and sensory impairments as well as attention deficit or hyperactivity disorders.

Trends in Mortality

The issue of using mortality data as a proxy for morbidity data was discussed previously in Chap. 2. To the extent that such proxy use is appropriate, data collected by the National Center for Health Statistics indicate steady improvement in the twentieth century in health status in terms of both mortality rates and life expectancy (National Center for Health Statistics 2015). The overall mortality rate for Americans in 2013 was age-adjusted 7.3 per 1000 population. This figure represents a decline from a rate of 25/1000 in 1900. In that year, the mortality rates for males and females were 26.3 and 24.1, respectively. The mortality rate for men declined from 15.9/1000 in 1970 to 8.6/1000 in 2013. For females, the mortality rate declined from 9.7 per 1000 to 6.2 per 1000 for this same period.

Life expectancy at birth and at age 65 increased steadily during the twentieth century, with life expectancy at birth 47.3 years in 1900 compared to 78.8 years in 2013. Life expectancy at birth for American males increased from 65.6 years in 1950 to 76.4 years in 2013 and for American females from 71.1 years to 81.2 years. Life expectancy at age 65 for males increased from 12.8 years to 17.9 years between 1950 and 2013 and for females from 15.0 years to 20.5 years.

The decline in mortality over the past century was essentially across the board—that is, impacting virtually all causes of death. However, some diseases contributed more heavily to the overall reduction in mortality while at least one disease recorded an increase in its contribution to mortality. Between 2000 and 2010, declines in death rates were reported for stroke (37 %), heart disease (30 %), cancer (16 %), and chronic lower respiratory disease (13 %). On the other hand, the death rate from Alzheimer's disease increased by 38 %. While observed changes in disease-specific death rates over time offers clues to trends in disease prevalence, the correlation between disease prevalence rates and mortality rates is far from perfect, especially when chronic conditions are being considered.

It should be noted that comparisons such as these often mask patterns of morbidity that are more complex. In the case of CHD, for example, a decline in the prevalence of this condition is suggested by the decrease in mortality from CHD between 1900 and 2010. However, in discussing the "decline and rise" of CHD Jones and Greene (2013) note that the trend toward a reduction in CHD mortality has actually reversed in the past 20 years. They argue that various factors have led to an uptick in the prevalence of CHD that on the one hand may represent a blip in the on-going trend toward improved health status or, on the other, indicate a definitive reversal of past trends. Similar patterns have been identified for other health conditions (e.g., certain infectious diseases), reminding us that we cannot take continued health improvement for granted nor can we assume that past trends automatically apply to future conditions.

Evidence such as that presented by Jones and Greene is supported by other observers who suggest that, although health status indicators like mortality rates and life expectancy have continued to improve, the rate of improvement appears to be slowing or even leveling off (Crimmins and Beltran-Sanchez 2011). Data collected by the National Center for Health Statistics indicate that overall mortality rates for Americans, while continuing to improve, were improving at a declining rate. Rates of decrease equaling as much as 10 % per year for crude birth rates prior to WWII dropped to 0.5 % per year for the 1970–2000 period and to 0.2 % for the 2000–2010 period. Age-adjusted death rates averaging declines of more than 10 % per year in the pre-war decades dropped to 0.16 % per year for the 1970–2000 period and to 0.07 % for 2000–2010 (Hoyert and Xu 2012).

While a slowing of the improvement in mortality rates was not unexpected, an actual increase in mortality rates was. In 2010 the overall age-adjusted mortality rate rose to 8.4/1000 compared to 8.2 in 2005. This reversal of the mortality trend, however, does not appear to be across the board but is driven by the adverse rates characterizing selected subgroups. Females appear to be most affected by this reversal, with female mortality rates in nearly half of US counties increasing between 1992 and 2006; only 3 % of counties saw male mortality increase over the same period (Kindig and Cheng 2013). It remains to be seen if this pattern is maintained or if this is a short-lived anomaly.

The most dramatic improvement in mortality rates, of course, has been for infant mortality, with most of the decline occurring during the first half of the twentieth century. Between 1900 and 2010 the maternal mortality rate dropped from around 80 per 1000 births in 1900 to 6.1 in 2010. As with the overall mortality rate, the rate of improvement slowed significantly after WWII. Between 1970 and 2000 the rate per 1000 live births dropped by an average of 0.4 per year. Between 2000 and 2010 the rate of improvement declined to half of that or 0.2 per year. The fact that the infant mortality rate continues to improve is encouraging but is offset by the decline in the rate of improvement.

As with other mortality rates, the maternal mortality rate declined rapidly during the first half of the twentieth century, with the rate of improvement slowing after WWII up until the 1980s. Death during childbirth in the US it seemed had been relegated, as they say, to the dustpan of history. However, unlike other mortality rates, the trend eventually began to reverse itself, hitting its lowest mark around 1980, stagnating during the 1980s and 1990s and actually increasing moving into the twenty-first century. The rate of less than 1.2 maternal deaths per 10000 live births in the 1980s increased to a modern high of nearly 2.5 deaths per 10000 live births in 2010. The rate has dropped slightly (to 1.85 in 2013) but the fact that the US is the only developed country in the world for which the maternal mortality rate is increasing is certainly noteworthy (Kassenbaum 2014).

Although life expectancy has continued to increase (although at an ever-slowing rate and at a rate lagging behind other developed countries), there is evidence of an actual *decline* in life expectancy among the poorly educated in the US (Olshansky et al. 2012). In his examination of Americans without a high school diploma it was found that life expectancy for white women without a high school diploma dropped 5 years between 1990 and 2008. A smaller decline of 3 years was found for white men over this period. It does not appear that uneducated whites are living shorter lives on the average but that many are being eliminated at younger ages. Thus, the life expectancy for white women without a high school diploma was 73.5 years in 2008 (compared to 83.9 years for women with a college degree) and for white men it was 67.5 years (compared to 80.4 years for those with a college degree). The fact that any segment of the US population is demonstrating a negative trend in mortality is worthy of note. Another study found that inequality in women's health outcomes steadily increased between 1985 and 2010, with female life expectancy stagnating or declining in 45 % of US counties (Wang et al. 2013). Recent research, thus, suggests that women in some parts of the country are dying younger than they were a generation ago.

Among the explanations that have been offered for adverse life expectancy trends are an increase in prescription drug overdoses, an increase in smoking, rising obesity, and a lack of health insurance. These factors appear to be particularly significant for women. The economic recession could be a contributor to observed trends, in combination with working in strenuous jobs while having children at a rate higher than the rest of the US population.

Given the body of data available on changing morbidity trends, the question arises as to whether the health status of Americans is continuing to improve or we are currently experiencing a reversal in morbidity fortunes. Exhibit 8.9 addresses the issue of whether the health of Americans is improving or declining.

Exhibit 8.9 Sicker or Healthier? Tracking the Level of Morbidity

An issue that is increasingly raised is whether Americans are becoming sicker or healthier than they used to be. While conventional wisdom suggests that we have steadily become healthier as a population over time, there is statistical evidence dating in some cases as far back as the 1980s to suggest otherwise. While it could be argued that more Americans are living longer, healthier lives than their ancestors, there is a growing body of evidence that the US population may be experiencing a reversal of health fortunes.

The answer to this question is complicated by the lack of a standard measure of morbidity. Researchers on this topic do not have access to any global indicator that they can point to. Aggregate measures (e.g., the combined prevalence of chronic conditions, overall disability) might be considered although there is likely to be disagreement over what diseases to include in any aggregate measure. Specific conditions could be considered (e.g., major health threats like heart disease and cancer, contributors to poor health such as obesity) but, again, there is likely to be disagreement over with conditions to include.

(continued)

Exhibit 8.9 (continued)

A common although subjective approach to determining the overall morbidity level is through the use of self-reported health status. Various surveys ask respondents to rate their health status on a scale from poor to excellent. The results on some surveys have indicated, in fact, a decline in the proportion of the US population rating their health as "very good" or "excellent," and an increase in the proportion rating their health as "poor" or "fair" between 1997 and 2010. This level of self-reported health status reflects a departure from the steadily increasing health status reported prior to 1997. These findings of decreasing health status are not consistent across all surveys, with a continued improvement in health status noted in some.

Other researchers have pointed to the steady increase in the prevalence of chronic disease within the US population. Of course, with the aging of the population, one should expect a decline in the incidence of acute conditions and an increase in the prevalence of chronic conditions. However, the prevalence rates for many chronic conditions are higher today for various older age groups than they were a generation ago, suggesting that more people are living longer but with more chronic conditions. Further, it is noted that certain acute conditions remain at epidemic levels (e.g., sexually transmitted infections) while many communicable diseases long eliminated if not eradicated from our population are making a comeback (e.g., measles, mumps, malaria).

Of particular concern are rising rates of noncommunicable chronic conditions such as obesity, diabetes, high blood pressure, heart disease, and cancer. In 2005, nearly half of adults—133 million—had at least one chronic illness. In 2009–2010, more than one-third (35.7 %) of US adults were obese, and 8.3 % had diabetes. In 2005–2008, over 30 % had high blood pressure. The prevalence of these conditions has grown substantially over the last 20 years and these trends are eroding previous advances the US made in life expectancy and other measures of population health. This notion is reinforced by the fact that a higher proportion of the population (in all age groups) is classified as disabled.

Of even more concern is the purported declining health status of America's children. The Institute of Medicine (IOM) reported in 2012 that "the current generation of children and young adults in the United States could become the first generation to experience shorter life spans and fewer healthy years of life than those of their parents." Of particular concern is the increase—driven to a great extent by the high and increasing rate of obesity—is the rise of chronic conditions among children. Conditions such as heart disease and diabetes were unknown among children in past generations but, along with other chronic conditions typically associated with the elderly, are becoming increasingly common.

(continued)

Exhibit 8.9 (continued)

Given all of the available evidence it is difficult to definitively conclude whether Americans are continuing to get healthy or are now becoming sicker. At the end of the day, the answer is probably: It depends. That is, depending on the metrics examined, the time period under consideration, and the population included, it is possible to end up with either result. However, the fact that a growing number of indicators suggest that Americans are becoming sicker is noteworthy. Clearly additional research is required to settle this issue.

References

Saloman, J. A., Nordhagen, S., Oza, S., & Murray, C. J. L. (2001). Are Americans feeling less healthy? The puzzle of trends in self-rated health. *American Journal of Epidemiology, 170*(3): 343–351.

Institute of Medicine. (2012). *For the public's health: Investing in a healthier future.* Retrieved from http://www.iom.edu/Reports/2012/For-the-Publics-Health-Investing-in-a-Healthier-Future.aspx.

Utilization as a Measure of Morbidity

Using trends in the utilization of health services as a proxy measure for morbidity is a complicated matter. As discussed in Chap. 5, the question is essentially whether high utilization rates indicate a high level of morbidity or, alternatively, a lower level of morbidity due to adequate access to care. While there is no shortage of data related to utilization, the challenge is in how to interpret it. The most likely answer again is: It depends. It depends on the type of utilization that is being measured and an understanding of the factors that contribute to health status.

Physician Visits

Physician office visits represent the most frequent form of formal healthcare utilization and might be deemed to reflect the level of morbidity within a population. The volume of visits and, importantly, the reasons for physician visits, should reflect the morbidity profile of the population. Baby boomers, for example, are visiting physicians at a higher rate than Americans in the same age cohort in previous periods. Between 1991 and 2011 the overall rate of physician visits increased from 2777/1000 population to 3004/1000. The visit rate to primary care providers remained the same during this period, while the visit rate to specialists increased. At the same time the visit rate for those under 45 was unchanged while the rate of physician utilization for older adults and seniors increased (National Center for Health Statistics 2013).

The observed increases are thought to be driven by aging baby boomers who require more frequent management/monitoring of chronic disease. Between 1996 and 2006 the number of physician office visits by those 55–64 increased by 13 % (Elliott 2010). Does this mean that "boomers" are sicker than their predecessors or that they are more health conscious or better insured? Increases in utilization rates for the population 45 years of age and over may be associated, in part, with greater emphasis on use of cholesterol- and glucose-lowering drugs which require monitoring by a physician, or on diagnostic testing such as mammography that consensus guidelines recommend commence after age 50. It should also be noted that Americans 65 years of age and over become eligible for Medicare coverage, which may improve access to physician care for people who were previously uninsured or under-insured.

Data available for a number of specific conditions provide insight into morbidity trends. While the visit rate for chronic obstructive pulmonary disease (COPD) decreased from 318 per 10000 population to 280 from 1992–1993 to 1999–2000, the rate of emergency department visits for COPD increased from 29/10000 to 44. Much of this increase can be attributed to higher rates for the oldest age cohorts (although increases were recorded for all age groups). The increase in visits to hospital, outpatient departments for all conditions exceeded the other indicators, growing from 15/10000 to 29/10000 over this period (perhaps reflecting the shift away from inpatient services).

The trend for diabetes has been even more clear-cut. While the physician office visit rate for patients with diabetes increased from 962/10000 to 1356/10000 between 1992–1993 and 1999–2000, reinforcing other data indicating an increase in the prevalence of diabetes. The emergency department visit rate for diabetes increased from 33 to 44 and the hospital admission rate jumped from 130 to 157 for this same period. The use rate for diabetes for hospital outpatient departments almost doubled during this period, from 84/10000 to 157/10000. Exhibit 8.10 discusses the confounding factor of geographic variations in utilization rates.

Overall utilization rates do not tell exactly what services are being provided to specific persons and cannot serve as proxies for either access to specific services or quality of care. A physician's office visit may include tests, procedures, and even surgery, or it may consist entirely of a discussion with a physician. A hospital or nursing home stay could be for diagnostic, palliative, or recuperative care, or for medical or surgical interventions. These trends can, however, spotlight areas that should be investigated in greater depth.

Exhibit 8.10 Geographic Variation in the Treatment of Health Conditions

Healthcare analysts long ago realized that significant variation exists in the utilization of health services from community to community in the United States. This is significant in that utilization (i.e., the number of reported cases) may be used as a proxy for the morbidity level. As early as the 1970s research revealed that the rate of procedures performed even in adjacent states varied to a degree not explained by population differences. The rate of performance of procedures could range from 10 % of the population in some markets to 50 % in others. These studies suggest that the level of health services utilization is less a function of disease prevalence than a reflection of the characteristics of the medical community and practice patterns of local physicians.

Typical of the findings on this issue are the results of a study that compared the cities of Boston and New Haven in terms of their health services utilization patterns. While the two cities were similar in terms of the factors that *should* determine the use of health services, they differed dramatically on virtually every indicator of health services utilization. The hospital admission rate, for example, was nearly twice as high in Boston as in New Haven. Furthermore, residents of Boston were much more likely to be hospitalized for various acute and chronic conditions than were residents of New Haven. The average annual per capita expenditure on healthcare in Boston was twice that of New Haven. However, the comparative utilization patterns were not always consistent. Certain procedures were performed much more frequently in Boston but others more frequently in New Haven.

It is now realized that a number of factors account for these seemingly inexplicable differences. A major factor is the variation in physician practice patterns from community to community. In some communities it is standard practice to treat a problem with surgery; in others the standard calls for less invasive treatment. In some communities conventional medical wisdom calls for hospitalization for certain diagnostic tests and procedures, whereas in others it is customary to handle such cases on an outpatient basis.

Other factors contributing to differential utilization rates include the relative supply of facilities and services. There is pressure, for example, to fill hospital beds if they are available and to use technology in which the organization has invested. In contrast to other industries, competition in healthcare often drives up both utilization levels and costs, thereby accounting for an additional degree of variation. Even the presence of a medical school may influence both the level of utilization and types of procedures performed. Increasingly, the level of managed care penetration is a significant factor influencing utilization rates.

Given these variations, how does the analyst know the appropriate level of utilization? Is the reported level of utilization high, low, or what should be

(continued)

Exhibit 8.10 (continued)

realistically expected? Of course, one way to address this is to use some standard measure such as the health services utilization rates developed by the National Center for Health Statistics based on national surveys. These rates provide useful benchmarks but, because most analyses focus on local markets, how appropriate are they for the community in question? There is no easy answer to this dilemma. The analyst must be able to gain enough knowledge about the local healthcare environment to make reasonable assessments about the level of utilization and the extent to which this reflects differences in actual prevalence rather than variations in medical practices.

Source: Wennberg, J. E., & Cooper, M. M. (Eds.). (1999). *The Dartmouth Atlas of Health Care*. Chicago: American Hospital Association.

Hospital Admissions

Hospital visits may be considered reflective of a population's morbidity profile in that they presumably involve more serious conditions. As with physician office visits, it is difficult to interpret trends in hospitalization when monitoring changes in morbidity. A number of factors influence the level of hospitalization again raising the key question: Is utilization a sign of poor health or good health? Hospital admission (or discharge) rates have declined significantly over the past quarter century, although the number of hospital admissions themselves has increased (American Hospital Association 2013). According to the National Center for Health Statistics (2013), the number of admissions was stable through the early 1990s but began increasing later in that decade. Some 38 million hospital admissions (to all hospitals) were recorded in 1980, reflecting a continuous upward trend since the end of WWII. This figure dropped to 34 million in 1990 and 33 million in 1995, no doubt reflecting the impact of the large relatively young (and healthy) baby boom cohort. Between 1995 and 2005 the upward trend was renewed, with admissions exceeding 37 million by 2005. Figures for 2010 suggest another moderation in this trend with less than 37 million admissions recorded. At the same time, the number of patient days recorded steadily dropped from 200 million in 1990 to barely 150 million in 2011 reflecting the decreasing average length of hospital stay (from age-adjusted 6.5 days in 1990 to 4.8 days in 2011). The ALOS has remained slightly under 5 days for at least a decade and is not likely to be reduced further in the future. Shorter lengths of stay, of course, do not necessarily translate into less sick patients; there are many other factors to consider.

Of more significance for this discussion is the hospital admission rate, which has experienced a steady decline over a quarter century. In 1980 the age-adjusted hospital admission rate was 174.4 per 1000 (or 17 % of the population in a given year), reflecting a continuous increase since the end of WWII. This figure declined steadily until 2000 (rate = 112.8/1000), followed by a spike around 2005 (117.4/1000). By 2011 the rate had returned to 112/1000 (National Center for Health Statistics 2013).

One could argue that the per capita decrease in hospital utilization reflects improving morbidity levels but it is difficult to accept this conclusion without serious reservations. Factors that influenced the level of hospital admission during this period include the shift from inpatient to outpatient care, the explosion in drug therapy, and restrictions placed on hospital admission by third-party payers. These significant developments make it risky to look at hospital admission rates in isolation from other measures. Now in the second decade of the twenty-first century, there are projections that aging baby boomers will generate an increase in hospital admissions for the foreseeable future. Contrary to expectations this development has not yet occurred and there are many factors that will eventually influence the level of hospital use.

Emergency Department and Hospital Outpatient Visits

The emergency department (ED) visit rate has not increased significantly since 1992 (the earliest available year of ED data), with rates between 356 and 394 visits per 1000 persons. At the same time, the rate for illness-related visits to EDs (as opposed to accidents) rose from 21.0 to 24.0 visits per 100 persons (Bernstein et al. 2003). It is hard to know how to interpret these figures, in that emergency department use may reflect a variety of factors that are unrelated to health status.

The number of hospital outpatient visits has increased dramatically, from 321 million in 1991 to 656 million in 2011 (American Hospital Association 2013). This reflects to a certain extent the shift of many inpatient services to the outpatient setting. This yields a rate increase from 1273/1000 population to 2106/1000. Between 1991 and 2011 the number of emergency department visits was up sharply, from 88 million to 130 million. This increase was reflected in the rate per 1000, with this figure increasing from 350/1000 in 1991 to 410/1000 in 2011.

Drug Prescription Rates

One other utilization measure that might be considered is the extent to which Americans are consuming prescription drugs. Here, the same question is raised as to whether high rates of "medicalization" represent high rates of disease or low rates of disease due to aggressive management. In this case, the argument probably goes to the former perspective, despite pressure from healthcare providers (spurred on by pharmaceutical companies) to aggressively diagnose and treat various conditions. Today, virtually no American (who can afford it) is not being "managed" to some extent through prescription drugs. Between 1996 and 2006, there was about a 25 % increase in the proportion of people receiving five or more prescriptions during a hospital visit. While the data on drug prescriptions written are abstracted from patient records at physicians' offices, there is no way of knowing whether the prescriptions were actually filled and/or the drugs consumed by the patient.

Data collected by the NCHS indicates increased rates of use (measured in terms of use within the past 30 days) between 1988/1994 and 2007/2010 for 14 of 15 classes of drugs. The most significant increases in utilization were recorded for cholesterol medications (735 % increase), antidepressants (483 %), anticonvulsants for epilepsy, seizures, and related conditions (285 %), blood pressure medication (beta blockers = 242 % and ACE inhibitors = 262 %), and antidiabetic medication (219 %). Increases in these categories were recorded for both males and females across the board. The 15 categories of drugs and their utilization trends are present in Exhibit 8.11 below.

Using diabetic drugs as an example, it was found that the rate of drug use increased between 1992–1993 and 1999–2000 from 20/1000 to around 50/1000 for those 18–44 years, from 140/1000 to over 200/1000 for those 45–64 years and from 300/1000 to over 500/1000 for those 65 years and older. These figures, of course, reflect data from those who actually presented themselves for treatment and do not take into account those who have not made office visits. However, it can be assumed that given the nature of the disease, these figures present a reasonably accurate measure to the extent of diagnosed diabetes within the population.

Exhibit 8.11: Trends in Utilization for Selected Prescription Drug Classes 1988/1994–2007/2010

Drug class	Percent of population with at least one prescription in past 30 days	
	1988/1994	2007/2010
Antihyperlipidemic agents	1.7	12.5
Analgesics	7.2	9.1
Antidepressants	1.8	8.7
Gastric reflux medication	2.8	8.6
Beta blockers	3.1	7.5
ACE inhibitors	2.4	6.3
Antidiabetic agents	2.6	5.7
Diuretics	3.4	5.3
Thyroid hormones	2.3	5.1
Bronchodilators	2.6	5.0
Sex hormones[a]	9.8	8.7
Anxiety medication	2.8	4.7
Antihypertension medication	2.4	4.5
Anticonvulsants	1.4	4.0
Calcium channel blocking agents	3.6	3.8

[a]Females only
Source: National Center for Health Statistics. (2013). Health United States 2012. Hyattsville, MD: National Center for Health Statistics.

Trends in the Factors Influencing Morbidity Change

While the factors that contribute to the morbidity profile are important and merit careful consideration, a detailed discussion of these factors is beyond the scope of this book. However, a brief review of the factors that are contributing to changing morbidity patterns is provided below.

Biologic Factors

Although biologic pathogens are considered to be a minor contributor to current morbidity patterns, there are some factors that will continue to provide etiologic contributions to the morbidity profile of the US population for the foreseeable future. One of the by-products of the successful treatment of common diseases has been the emergence of new, drug-resistant strains of pathogens. Bacteria, viruses, fungi, and protozoa all can produce mutations that are not amenable to treatment by previously effective drugs (Michael et al. 2014). The overuse of antibiotics is considered a major consideration in the rise of drug-resistant pathogens.

Another development to consider is the reemergence of certain communicable diseases that were eliminated if not eradicated during the twentieth century (National Institute of Allergy and Infectious Diseases 2015). As discussed earlier in this chapter, reduced efforts on the part of public health officials (typically due to lack of funding) have led to the reappearance of certain diseases within the population that were thought to belong to a past era. In addition, the misguided anti-vaccine "movement" has also contributed to the reemergence of diseases such as whooping cough, mumps, and measles. Unsuccessful efforts toward the control of common infectious disease (such as sexually transmitted infections) have resulted in something of an epidemic of infectious diseases. Finally, the flow of immigrants into the US from countries where communicable diseases are still common has led to the reintroduction of certain diseases.

The immigration flow mentioned above is also considered to be a factor in the introduction of *new* communicable diseases (National Institute of Allergy and Infectious Diseases 2015). These are diseases that may be common elsewhere in the world but have not historically affected the US population. While the impact of new diseases introduced via immigration is considered minimal in the overall morbidity profile, the continued "shrinking" of the world can be expected to continue to put the US population at some risk for exposure to new diseases.

Environmental Factors

Changes in both the natural and social (built) environment will continue to affect the US morbidity profile. The modification of the natural environment is a global phenomenon, and human activity in even far-flung regions of the world has implications for the US population and its health status. Human actions are contributing to the changes in the natural environment as we continue to pollute our air, water, and land. These activities affect the status of plants and animals in our environment which in turn affect our health. Extractive activities have documented adverse effects on our land and water which ultimately affect our food supply. These factors affect the health status of those with direct exposure as well as those indirectly affected "downstream." Americans who reside close to toxic waste dumps experience higher rates of disease (U.S. Environmental Protection Agency 2015), and we are only now beginning to understand the impact of "fracking" on our health (Physicians for Social Responsibility 2015).

There is increasing documentation of current and potential impact of climate change on human health. Although the US population may be more insulated from the effects of climate change than many other populations, the effects will only be delayed and the CDC is beginning to warn of potential health threats. The direct effects are being felt now with erratic and often violent weather conditions. The indirect results of these phenomena are changed conditions for agriculture that may ultimately affect the food supply. Some of the factors that are contributing to climate—such as environmental degradation and loss of habitat for flora and fauna—have health implications of their own.

The built environment in the US also carries certain health threats. The loss of green space and increased congestion both have implications for the health of the population. Urban concentrations create "heat islands" that can be detrimental to health and a lack of green space is associated with poor health status (Hunter et al. 2015). We are only now beginning to understand the impact of various policies and projects on the health of the affected populations.

Social Structural Effects

A number of aspects of social structure have implications for health status and, in the short run, may be more of a factor than environmental threats. Perhaps the most immediate and far-reaching aspect of US social structure is the growing economic inequality accompanied by poverty rates that were thought to have been left behind 30 years ago. As resources (including healthcare) become more concentrated in fewer and fewer hands the opportunities for benefiting from these resources are denied to more and more people. The disparities observed in health status between various segments of the population, while moderated somewhat in recent years, remain at unacceptably high levels. The inequalities that exist extend to access to health services, to green space, to safe environments and to healthy foods, contributing to the unfavorable health status of much of the population. Even access to education has an indirect impact on health status as those with limited education face higher health risks and, now, a documented greater risk of mortality (Wang et al. 2013).

The availability of health services is a structural consideration that is often overlooked. Despite the US reputation for ample healthcare resources—especially technology—the distribution of these resources is very uneven. Health resources are increasingly concentrated in fewer and fewer locations, often leaving residents of rural areas and urban cores without access to basic services much less specialty care and advanced technology. Even with access to health insurance (see below) the health status of those who face physical, social, or cultural barriers to healthcare access may be adversely affected. The maldistribution and even shortages for some healthcare resources are likely to persist for the foreseeable future.

Another "structural" consideration is the availability of health insurance for the population. Until recently as many as 50 million Americans lacked health insurance coverage, despite evidence of the correlation between insurance coverage and both health status and mortality risk. The enactment of the Affordable Care Act in 2010 has contributed to an improvement in this situation, although millions continue to fall through the cracks with regard to insurance coverage. Here again, access to insurance does not guarantee access to care and the ultimate impact of expanded coverage has yet to be determined.

Demographics

It could be argued that demographics is destiny when it comes to US morbidity patterns. The epidemiologic transition that the US has been experiencing for the past quarter century may be the single most important factor affecting the future morbidity profile. The changing age structure augers continued changes in the nature of the health problems, with acute conditions giving way to chronic conditions. These developments do not necessarily predict more health problems—although there will clearly be more temporarily as the baby boomers cycle through—but certainly different health problems. Not only will the typical patient be older than they are today but the patient will more likely to be female with all the implications that carries.

The increasing racial and ethnic diversity will also contribute to the changing morbidity picture. Different racial and ethnic groups exhibit different health status profiles and often suffer from group-specific health conditions. Members of all groups except non-Hispanic whites tend to be younger than the average and can be expected to exhibit a higher incidence of acute conditions. As the population becomes more diverse it could be argued for a bifurcated morbidity picture with an older white population affected by chronic disease and a younger population of African-Americans, Hispanics, Asian-Americans and other minority groups characterized as least for a period by acute conditions.

Changes in household and family structure may also carry implications for health status. The fact that fewer and fewer Americans live in "traditional" families may have implications for health status. Historically it has been found that those who are married tend to have higher health status than those in other marital status categories.

Further, those in stable households also exhibit more favorable health status. It could be argued, therefore, that these trends suggest a higher level of morbidity in the future for these populations. Those living in single-parent households—the fastest growing household type—appear to be particularly susceptible to health problems.

Changing income and educational levels also have implications for health status. Historically, as income levels and educational attainment have increased, so has the population's health status. To the extent that the US median household income and median educational attainment continue to rise, one could argue for improved health status and declining morbidity. While this could happen, the increasing inequality in both income and education observed for the US population may have a mitigating impact on anticipated improvements in health status. A consequence of increased inequality in income and education is greater variation in both access to care and "health literacy." Thus, while one portion of the population is likely to benefit from increasing incomes and educational attainment, large segments of the population may experience the opposite effect—that is, declining health status.

Lifestyles

Most observers argue that the lifestyles presently engaged in by the US population are the major contributor to the current morbidity profile. Dietary patterns, physical activity and involvement in either health-favorable or health-unfavorable behaviors are major factor when we consider future morbidity patterns. Americans have become addicted to the types of foods that contribute to poor health, and, despite the fitness "craze" they tend to get less exercise than previous generations. Increased obesity levels for adults and children have probably had as great an impact on the changing morbidity profile as has the aging of the population. Although tobacco use has declined, alcohol and drug abuse are rampant, contributing to higher rates for certain health problems. While the lifestyles that most Americans follow today tend to be detrimental to health, there are subgroups within the population that pursue lifestyles that are even more hazardous to their health, not only involving poor diet and exercise habits but involving drug, tobacco and alcohol abuse and risky sexual behavior.

Medical Science/Healthcare Developments

Although the role of formal medical care has been accorded limited credit for the changes that have occurred in US morbidity patterns, it would be inappropriate to not consider the role of the healthcare system in the emerging morbidity profile. Clearly, the US healthcare system can relatively efficiently address diseased individuals, providing a level of care unrivaled elsewhere. However, it could be argued, the impact of the healthcare system (public health excluded) typically occurs after the fact. Its strong point is the system's ability to fix things once they are broken. What the system is not good at is preventing health problems in the first place. For this reason, it could be argued, the formal healthcare system is not going to have much of an impact on future morbidity patterns unless or until it adopts a population health approach.

In the meantime, the one component of the healthcare system that does impact overall health status is public health. In fact, most of the improvement in the health status of Americans has been credited to public health (along with changing demographic attributes), rather than to "private" medicine. Public health already represents a form of population health and to the extent that it addresses broad population issues rather than individual patient needs, it represents a better candidate for affecting future morbidity patterns. However, there are concerns about the declining influence of public health as funding issues and ideological considerations are limiting the impact of public health efforts. While activities that come under the umbrella of public health have much better chance of affecting the future health status of the population, the unstable funding situation may limit the impact of public health efforts to improve health status.

Governmental Intervention

One final consideration is the impact of government intervention on future morbidity patterns. Historically, governments at all levels have had little relative impact on the health status profile of the population. While it could be argued that the public health function represents government intervention, this is true only to a certain point. Public health authorities have little ability to enforce programs on the general population (except in the case of serious public health threats), and public health represents the most direct role that government plays in this regard.

It could be argued that the role the government plays in the healthcare system through its support of the Medicare and Medicaid programs is a factor in determining the level of morbidity within the population. While these programs have an impact on the types of health services that are provided and utilized, their impact is really after the fact—that is, after the morbid conditions have been established within the population. At the very best, the role of government in these programs may have an impact on morbidity patterns by virtue of the treatment provided (and much more minimally) through prevention-oriented programs.

The government may also have influence through the operation of various programs through departments that are not primarily health oriented. The Environmental Protection Agency, the Department of Labor and the Department of Agriculture, for example, all support programs that have the potential to influence the health status of the population. A more relevant example may even be the Food and Drug Administration. While these agencies offer some programs that may have a relatively direct impact on the health of the population (e.g., drug approval, food inspection, workplace safety), the overall effect is likely to be limited relative to the broader role of demographics and lifestyles in determining morbidity patterns. In today's ideological environment, there is considerable resistance to even the limited role that government plays in improving our health status. When the First Lady of the United States is ridiculed for supporting healthy food for school children it is clear that any government—especially the federal government—is not likely to have much direct impact on the health status of the population.

References

Adams, D., Jajosky, R. A., Agani, U., et al. (2014). *Summary of notifiable diseases—United States, 2012*. Retrieved from http://www.cdc.gov/mmwr/preview/mmwrhtml/mm6153a1.htm.

American Hospital Association. (2013). Chapter 3: Utilization and volume. *Trends affecting hospitals and health systems*. Retrieved from http://www.aha.org/research/reports/tw/chartbook/2014/chapter3.pdf.

Armour, B. (2010). The importance of paying attention to the health of people with disabilities. Retrieved from http://www.aucd.org/docs/ncbddd/Brian%20Armour.pdf.

Bailey, J. (2014). *The end of healing*. Memphis, TN: The Healthy City Press.

Bernstein, A. B., Hing, E., Moss, A. J., Allen, K. F., Siller, A. B., & Tiggle, R. B. (2003). *Health care in America: Trends in utilization*. Hyattsville, MD: National Center for Health Statistics.

Boyle, J. P. (2010). Projection of the year 2050 burden of diabetes in the US adult population: Dynamic modeling of incidence, mortality, and prediabetes prevalence. *Population Health Metrics, 8*, 29.

Crimmins, E. M., & Beltran-Sanchez, H. (2011). Mortality and morbidity trends: Is there compression of morbidity? *Journal of Gerontology and Psychological Social Science, 66B*(1), 75–86.

Delaney, L., & Smith, J. P. (2012). Childhood health: Trends and consequences over the life course. *The Future of Children, 22*(1), 43–63.

Dohrenwend, B. P., & Dohrenwend, B. S. (1974). Social and cultural influences on psychopathology. *Annual Review of Psychology, 25*, 417–447.

Dohrenwend, B. P., et al. (1980). *Mental illness in the United States: Epidemiological estimates*. New York: Praeger.

Elliott, V. S. (2010). Older baby boomers sicker, using more care than earlier generations. *American Medical News*. Retrieved from http://www.amednews.com/article/20100419/business/304199954/6/.

Federal Interagency Forum on Aging-Related Statistics. (2004). *Older Americans, 2004*. Retrieved from http://www.agingstats.gov/agingstatsdotnet/Main_Site/Data/2004_Documents/entire_report.pdf.

Feigin, V. L., Forouzanfar, M. H., Krishnamurthi, R., et al. (2014). Global and regional burden of stroke during 1990–2010: Findings from the Global Burden of Disease Study 2010. *The Lancet, 383*(9913), 245–254.

Freid, V. M., Bernstein, A. B., & Bush, M. A. (2012, July). *Multiple chronic conditions among adults aged 45 and over: trends over the past 10 years*. (NCHS Data Brief No. 100).

Hall, J. P., Kurth, N. K., & Fall, E. C. (2012). Discrepancy among behavioral risk factor surveillance system, social security, and functional disability measurement. *Disability and Health Journal, 5*, 60–63.

Hedden, S., Gfroerer, J., & Barker, P., et al. (2012). Comparison of NSDUH mental health data and methods with other data sources. *CBHSQ Data Review*. Retrieved from http://www.samhsa.gov/data/sites/default/files/2k12Findings/2k12Findings/CBHSQDataReviewC2MentalHealth2012.htm.

Hoyert, L., & Xu, J. (2012). *Deaths: Preliminary data from 2012*. Retrieved from http://www.cdc.gov/nchs/data/nvsr/nvsr61/nvsr61_06.pdf.

Hunter, R., et al. (2015). The impact of interventions to promote physical activity in urban green space: A systematic review and recommendations for future research. *Social Science & Medicine, 124*, 246–256.

Institute of Medicine. (2006). *The future of disability in America*. Washington, DC: Institute of Medicine.

Institute of Medicine. (2012). *For the public's health: investing in a healthier future*. Retrieved from http://www.iom.edu/Reports/2012/For-the-Publics-Health-Investing-in-a-Healthier-Future.aspx.

Jones, D. S., & Greene, J. A. (2013). The decline and rise of coronary heart disease: Understanding public health catastrophism. *American Journal of Public Health, 103*, 1207–1218.

Kassenbaum, N. J. (2014, May 2). *Global, Regional, and National Levels and Causes of Maternal Mortality during 1990–2013: A Systematic Analysis for the Global Burden of Disease Study 2013*. Lancet. Retrieved from http://download.thelancet.com/flatcontentassets/pdfs/S0140673614604979.pdf.

Kessler, R. C., Chiu, W. T., Demler, O., et al. (2005). Prevalence, severity, and Comorbidity of twelve-month DSM-IV disorders in the National Comorbidity Survey Replication (NCS-R). *Archives of General Psychiatry, 62*(6), 617–627.

Kindig, D. A., & Cheng, E. R. (2013). Even as mortality fell in most US counties, female mortality nonetheless rose in 42.8 percent of counties from 1992 to 2006. *Health Affairs, 32*(3), 451–458.

MEDTAP International. (2004). *The value of investment in healthcare*. Retrieved from http://www.aha.org/content/00-10/Value_Report.pdf.

Michael, C. A., Dominey-Howes, D., & Labbate, M. (2014). The antimicrobial resistance crisis: Causes, consequences, and management. *Frontiers in Public Health, 2*, 145.

Mojtabai, R. (2011). National trends in mental health disability, 1997–2009. *American Journal of Public Health, 101*(11), 2156–2163.

Morrisey, M. (2015). Are disability rates increasing? Retrieved from http://www.epi.org/blog/are-disability-rates-increasing/.

National Center for Health Statistics. (2008). *Health: United States, 2007*. Hyattsville, MD: National Center for Health Statistics.

National Center for Health Statistics. (2012). *Health: United States, 2013*. Hyattsville, MD: National Center for Health Statistics.

National Center for Health Statistics. (2013). *Health: United States, 2012*. Hyattsville, MD: National Center for Health Statistics.

National Center for Health Statistics (2015). Deaths: Final data for 2013. Retrieved from http://www.cdc.gov/nchs/data/nvsr/nvsr64/nvsr64_02.pdf.

National Institute of Allergy and Infectious Diseases. (2015). Emerging infectious diseases/pathogens. Retrieved from http://www.niaid.nih.gov/topics/emerging/pages/introduction.aspx.

Nauert, R. (2010). Diagnostic trends in mental health. *Psych Central*. Retrieved from http://psych-central.com/news/2010/03/29/diagnostic-trends-in-mental-health/12411.html.

Newacheck, P. W., Budetti, P. P., & McManus, P. (1984). Trends in childhood disability. *American Journal of Public Health, 74*(3), 232–236.

Nihiser, A. J., Wechsler, H., McKenna, M., et al. (2004). Body mass index measurement in schools. *Journal of School Health, 77*(10), 651–671.

Olshansky, S. J., Antonucci, T., Berkman, L., et al. (2012). Differences in life expectancy Due to race and educational differences are widening, and many may not catch Up. *Health Affairs, 31*(8), 1803–1813.

Pal, S. (2011). Trends in mental health disorders. *U.S. Pharmacist*. Retrieved from http://www.uspharmacist.com/content/c/31041/?t=men's_health,psychotropic_disorders.

Physicians for Social Responsibility. (2015). Hydraulic fracking: How great is the danger to health? Retrieved from http://www.psr.org/environment-and-health/environmental-health-policy-institute/hydraulic-fracking.html.

Saloman, J. A., Nordhagen, S., Oza, S., & Murray, C. J. L. (2001). Are Americans feeling less healthy? The puzzle of trends in self-rated health. *American Journal of Epidemiology, 170*(3), 343–351.

U.S. Census Bureau. (2015). Disability statistics. Retrieved from https://www.disabilitystatistics.org/reports/acs.cfm?statistic=1.

U.S. Environmental Protection Agency. (2015). Hazardous substances and hazardous waste. Retrieved from http://www.epa.gov/superfund/students/clas_act/haz-ed/ff_01.htm.

Wang, P. S., Olfson, L. M., Pincus, H. A., et al. (2005). Twelve month use of mental health services in the United States. *Archives of General Psychiatry, 62*(6), 629–640.

Wang, H., Schumacher, A. E., Carly, E. L., et al. (2013). Left behind: Widening disparities for males and females in US county life expectancy, 1985–2010. *Population Health Metrics, 11*, 8.

Ward, B. W., Schiller, J. S., & Goodman, R. A. (2014). Multiple chronic conditions among US adults: a 2012 update. *Preventing Chronic Disease, 11:*130389. doi:http://dx.doi.org/10.5888/pcd11.130389.

Wennberg, J. E., & Cooper, M. M. (Eds.). (1999). *The Dartmouth Atlas of Health Care*. Chicago: American Hospital Association.

Chapter 9
Sources of Morbidity Data

Introduction

Once familiar with the morbidity data available, the challenge becomes one of finding and accessing appropriate data sources. It should be remembered that, unlike the case for fertility and mortality data, there is no one source for morbidity data. Neither is there one source that generates or aggregates data on sickness and disability nor any central repository of morbidity data. As a result health data users are required to draw from a variety of sources, with the resource accessed depending on the needs of the researcher. This situation, of course, creates a number of issues for those seeking to utilize morbidity data, especially when data are required from disparate sources. Morbidity data drawn from federal sources (e.g., the National Center for Health Statistics) may not be compatible with data drawn from private sources (e.g., health insurance plans, health system repositories) or even with data from other government sources (e.g., state hospital data repositories). These issues are highlighted as appropriate in the sections that follow.

For our purposes the sources of morbidity data have been grouped into the categories of government sources, association sources, and private industry sources. While this grouping is somewhat clumsy in that there is some overlap between the categories and not every source fits neatly into one or the other of the categories, this appeared to be the most systematic approach to take. This information is followed by a discussion of the synthetic data (i.e., estimates and projections) that are generated to fill gaps in existing morbidity data.

© Springer New York 2016
R.K. Thomas, *In Sickness and In Health*, Applied Demography Series 6,
DOI 10.1007/978-1-4939-3423-2_9

Sources of Morbidity Data

Government Sources

Governments at all levels are involved in the generation, compilation, manipulation, and/or dissemination of health-related data. The federal government is the world's largest processor of health-related data, including data on morbidity. Through the Centers for Disease Control and Prevention, the National Center for Health Statistics, the National Institutes for Health, and other agencies within the federal government, a large share of the nation's health data is generated. Federal agencies not generally associated with health data, such as the Department of Education (e.g., obesity among school children) and the Department of Agriculture (e.g., nutritional levels), directly or indirectly generate morbidity data. Federal sources are discussed in more detail below.

State and local governments are also sources of health-related data. State governments may generate some morbidity data, with each state having a different set of health factors to consider. State health departments theoretically compile data on morbidity but this is typically not done in a comprehensive manner and is not consistent from state to state. Although statistics on mortality can be obtained at the state level, mortality data, as noted earlier, do not necessarily serve as a proxy for morbidity data. State health departments do collect data on notifiable diseases (as do local health departments) but beyond that the type of morbidity data will vary from state to state, depending on the responsibilities of the respective state agency. State health departments may collect data on such diverse measures of morbidity as birth defects, exposure to environmental toxins, obesity, mental retardation, and a variety of other conditions. Thus, the ability to access data on a particular aspect of morbidity will vary from state to state. Researchers may also face situations where data from state agencies are not available below the state level or, at the very least below the county level, creating barriers to certain types of analyses.

Government agencies collect morbidity data through a variety of mechanisms. These include on-going surveillance systems (e.g., the Centers for Disease Control and Prevention), registration systems that track specific conditions (e.g., the CDC, state agencies), administrative records that reflect morbidity-related encounters or transactions (e.g., Medicare utilization data), and sample surveys (e.g., the National Center for Health Statistics). The agencies involved in these activities, their data collection and dissemination methods, and the relative usefulness of the various sources are noted below.

Federal Data Sources

Centers for Disease Control and Prevention Data Collection Programs

The Centers for Disease Control and Prevention (CDC) have been involved in disease-surveillance activities since the establishment of the Communicable Disease Center in 1946. Its initial responsibility involved the study of malaria, murine typhus, smallpox, and other communicable diseases. Surveillance activities now include programs in human reproduction, environmental health, chronic disease, risk reduction, occupational safety and health, and infectious diseases.

The CDC collects morbidity data through two main mechanisms: (1) on-going surveillance activities and (2) sample surveys. The most comprehensive set of morbidity data from the CDC involves notifiable diseases. By definition, the list of notifiable diseases is essentially restricted to communicable diseases, thereby omitting chronic conditions for all practical purposes. In the past three decades, however, chronic conditions (along with behavioral and lifestyle-caused diseases) have come to be the main factors in both morbidity and mortality for the US population, and efforts are being made on the part of the CDC to expand their monitoring of chronic conditions. Statistics on notifiable diseases are published weekly by the CDC in *Morbidity and Mortality Weekly Report* (MMWR) and compiled in other publications of the agency.

The CDC conducts national surveys that collect data on a wide range of factors including morbidity. Although labeled as "surveillance systems," these initiatives are survey based. The two major surveys for our purposes involve the Behavioral Risk Factor Surveillance System (BRFSS) and the Youth Risk Behavior Surveillance System (YRBSS). The BRFSS was initiated in 1995 to collect information on the health behavior and lifestyles of the US population. The survey includes data collection on such timely items as smoking, alcohol and drug use, seat belt use, and obesity, as well as other factors that might contribute to one's health status profile. Importantly, it includes items on disease prevalence and collects self-reported data on a variety of health conditions. Many of the items relate to chronic conditions, since these are not monitored through the standard surveillance mechanisms, and to behavioral health conditions for which there is no on-going monitoring system.

The YRBSS involves a national school-based survey conducted by the Centers for Disease Control and Prevention (CDC) and state, territorial, tribal, and local surveys conducted by state, territorial, and local education and health agencies and tribal governments. Through the YRBSS the CDC monitors priority health-risk behaviors and the prevalence of obesity and asthma among youth and young adults. Examples of additional CDC surveillance activities are presented in Exhibit 9.1.

Exhibit 9.1: Surveillance Activities Generating Morbidity Data

Tuberculosis Surveillance. The Tuberculosis Surveillance system compiles data on TB cases collected from 59 reporting areas (the 50 states, the District of Columbia, New York City, US dependencies and possessions, and independent nations in free association with the United States). Data from the system can be accessed through Online Tuberculosis Information System (OTIS), a query-based system containing information on verified tuberculosis (TB) cases reported to the Centers for Disease Control and Prevention (CDC).

Pediatric Nutrition Surveillance. The Pediatric Nutrition Surveillance System (PedNSS) is a program-based surveillance system that monitors the nutritional status of low-income infants, children, and women in federally funded maternal and child health programs. PedNSS data represent nearly

(continued)

Exhibit 9.1 (continued)

eight million children from birth to age 5. PNSS data are abstracted from approximately 1.3 million pregnant and postpartum women.

Pregnancy Surveillance System. The Pregnancy Surveillance System (PNSS) collects health data on a nationwide sample of mothers and their children. Surveillance data available at this site include national data tables with contributor-specific data on health indicators. This system generates data that describe prevalence of and trends in nutrition, health, and behavioral indicators.

National Diabetes Surveillance System (NDSS). The NDSS tracks cases of diabetes nationwide in order to measure the public health burden of diabetes and its complications. The Diabetes Indicators and Data Sources Internet Tool (DIDIT) is a user-friendly web-based tool designed to support surveillance, epidemiology, and program evaluation activities of state diabetes control programs.

National Oral Health Surveillance System (NOHSS). The NOHSS is a collaborative effort between CDC's Division of Oral Health and the Association of State and Territorial Dental Directors (ASTDD). NOHSS is designed to monitor the burden of oral disease, the use of the oral healthcare delivery system, and the status of community water fluoridation on both a national and state level. NOHSS is designed to track oral health surveillance indicators based on data sources and surveillance capacity at the state level.

National Biomonitoring Program (NBP). The NBP within the CDC's Environmental Health Laboratory assesses the level of exposure to toxic substances in the environment by measuring the substances or their metabolites in human specimens, such as blood and urine. Biomonitoring measurements are the most health-relevant assessments of exposure because they indicate the amount of the chemical that actually gets into people from all environmental sources.

Disability and Health Data System (DHDS). The Disability and Health Data System collects state-level, disability-specific health data. DHDS data based on findings from the Behavioral Risk Factor Surveillance System (BRFSS). It includes 79 health and demographic indicators stratified by disability status, 49 indicators stratified by psychological distress, and over 79 different health and demographic indicators for people with, and without, disabilities.

National Center for HIV/AIDS, Viral Hepatitis, STD, and TB Surveillance (NCHHSTP). The NCHHSTP tracks a number of communicable conditions and makes data on these conditions available at the NCHHSTP metrics dashboard. Trends in the incidence of these highly contagious conditions and data on the characteristics of affected persons are available at the state level.

National Center for Health Statistics Data Collection

Through the National Center for Health Statistics, the federal government administers a number of on-going surveys that deal with hospital utilization, ambulatory care utilization, nursing home and home health utilization, medical care expenditures, and other relevant topics. One of the Center's responsibilities includes the compilation, analysis, and publication of vital statistics for the United States and each relevant subarea. This function provides the basis for the calculation of fertility and mortality rates. The compilation and analysis of data on morbidity is another important function, and the Center has been responsible for the development of much of the epidemiological data available on chronic diseases.

The sample surveys conducted by the NCHS are generally large scale and fall into two categories: community-based surveys and facility-based surveys. Perhaps the Center's most important survey for our purposes is the National Health Interview Survey (NHIS), in which data are collected annually from approximately 49000 households. The NHIS is a key source of data on the incidence/prevalence of health conditions, health status, the number of injuries and disabilities characterizing the population, health services utilization, and a variety of other health-related topics. Other surveys that involve a sample from the community include the Medical Expenditure Panel Survey (MEPS), the National Health and Nutrition Examination Survey (NHANES), and the National Survey of Family Growth (NSFG). Another survey, the National Maternal and Infant Health Survey (NMIHS), involves a sampling of certificates of birth, fetal death, and infant death. While none of these surveys is devoted exclusively to the collection of morbidity data, each contributes to our knowledge of morbidity in its own way.

The NCHS is a major source of data on specific conditions, particularly important conditions such as chronic diseases that are not tracked by its parent organization the CDC. These data may be available through disease-specific online applications or portals. Examples of these sources include the Web-Based Injury Statistics Query and Reporting System (WISQARS), an interactive database system that provides customized reports of injury-related data from the National Center of Health Statistics (NCHS) and the violent death rate.

Summary data for specific conditions can be easily accessed via the NCHS website, with links provided to more detailed data. Exhibit 9.2 presents an excerpt from a web page from the NCHS site.

Exhibit 9.2: Crude and Age-Adjusted Rate per 100 of Civilian, Noninstitutionalized Population with Diagnosed Diabetes, United States, 1980–2011

From 1980 through 2011, the crude prevalence of diagnosed diabetes increased 176 % (from 2.5 to 6.9 %). During this period, increases in the crude and age-adjusted prevalence of diagnosed diabetes were similar, indicating that most of the increase in prevalence was not because of changes in the population age structure.

(continued)

Exhibit 9.2 (continued)

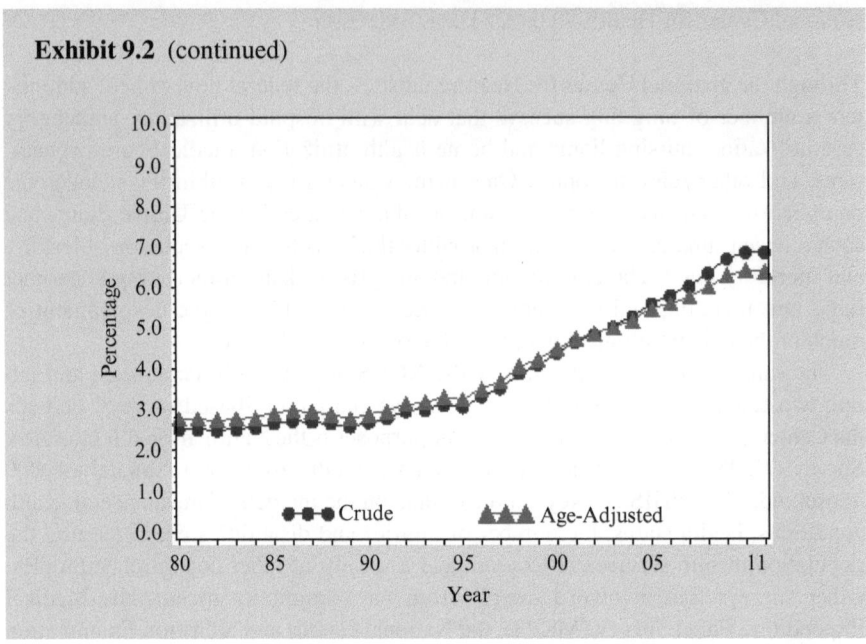

The data collected through NCHS studies are disseminated in a variety of ways. Some of the information is still disseminated as printed material, although "hard copies" are becoming less and less available. The Center's publications include annual books such as *Health, United States* (the "official" government compendium of statistics on the nation's health), and periodicals such as *Vital and Health Statistics*. Increasingly, data and reports generated by the NCHS are only available online. NCHS surveys have been described in previous chapters and the major ones that generate morbidity-related data are listed in Exhibit 9.3.

Exhibit 9.3: Major NCHS Surveys

- The *National Health Interview Survey* (NHIS) is an ongoing national survey of the US population and the data gathered generate information on demographic characteristics, physician visits, hospital stays, restricted-activity days, disability status, health status, and chronic conditions.
- The *Current Population Survey* (CPS) gathers detailed demographic data and information on health issues and insurance coverage for the US population.
- The *National Hospital Care Survey* (NHCS) is a new survey that combines the National Hospital Discharge Survey with surveys on emergency department use, outpatient visits, and hospital-based ambulatory care. Information is collected on the demographic, clinical, and financial characteristics of patients utilizing any of these forms of care.

(continued)

Exhibit 9.3 (continued)

- The *National Ambulatory Medical Care Survey* (NAMCS) is a nationwide survey designed to provide information about the provision and utilization of ambulatory health services. Demographic data on patients at physician offices are gathered, along with the reason for the visit, expected source(s) of payment, principle diagnosis, diagnostic services provided, and the disposition of the visit.
- The *National Nursing Home Survey* (NNHS) is a periodically conducted national survey of nursing and related care homes, their residents, their discharges, and their staffs.
- The *National Home and Hospice Care Survey* (NHHCS), last conducted in 2007, involves the collection of data from a sample of 1200 home health agencies and hospices. Patient questionnaires were administered for the various agencies and information was collected on the demographic and health characteristics of the patients served by these agencies.
- The *National Survey of Family Growth* (NSFG) collects data on factors affecting birth and pregnancy rates, adoption, and maternal and infant health, including information on sexual activity, contraception and sterilization practices, infertility, pregnancy loss, low birth-weight, and the use of medical care for family planning.
- Medical Expenditure Panel Survey (MEPS) is designed to generate data on the types, frequency, and costs related to medical services, including information on health insurance coverage.

To the extent that utilization data can be used as a proxy for morbidity data, the NCHS is the major source of such information. Primarily through its various surveys the NCHS collects data on hospital admissions, emergency department visits, outpatient procedures, physician office visits, and other measures of utilization. Often these encounters are categorized in terms of the diseases represented. Thus, it is possible to track the volume of physician visits over time, the most frequent reasons for hospital admission, and the characteristics of those using emergency department services. Much of this information can be accessed online from the Center's FastStats resource (as in the example in Exhibit 9.4). Links are provided to websites and/or publications that provide more detailed data. The NCHS electronic publication *Health, United States* serves as a compendium for much of the information drawn from NCHS surveys.

Exhibit 9.4: Physician Office Visits Summary United States 2010

- Number of visits: 1.0 billion
- Number of visits per 100 persons: 332.2
- Percent of visits made to primary care physicians: 55.5 %
- Most frequent principal illness-related reason for visit: cough
- Most commonly diagnosed condition: essential hypertension

Source: National Ambulatory Medical Care Survey: 2010.

Other Federal Sources

The 28 institutes that constitute the National Institutes of Health (NIH) represent another source of morbidity data. Each Institute tracks the incidence/prevalence rates of diseases under its purview and makes information on trends and affected populations available. Each Institute has its own approach to data collection and dissemination, and it may take some investigation to find the data related to a particular disease. It is beyond the scope of this discussion to list all of the data sources available through NIH components. However, it should be noted that the various Institutes are very inconsistent in their data dissemination approaches and, in some cases, it may not be possible to easily determine the types of data that an Institute has available.

The Centers for Medicare and Medicaid Services (CMS) collect a voluminous amount of data through the management of their beneficiaries' health claims. The quality and accessibility of the Medicare data is better than that for Medicaid since the former is centrally administered and the latter is complicated by a variety of state-specific models whose data are administered through intermediaries. Thus, detailed Medicare data is more likely to be available than comparable Medicaid data. Data generated by CMS primarily involves utilization data which can be used as a proxy for incidence/prevalence with the caveats previously noted.

The Agency for Healthcare Research and Quality (AHRQ) sponsors research on a variety of health topics and conducts its own research on certain topics. While most AHRQ-sponsored research is not specifically focused on morbidity, it does collect a significant amount of utilization data that might serve as a proxy for morbidity data. AHRQ also collaborates with other agencies such as the NIH in conducting research, integrating findings, and disseminating data.

State Sources of Morbidity Data

States represent an important source of morbidity data, some of which is only available at the state level. While the collection of morbidity data is typically not a stated function of most state agencies, a considerable amount of data is collected in the course of agency operation. State health departments are understandably an important source of health-related data. All states generate mortality statistics and in a form that allows for state-to-state comparisons. To the extent that mortality data can be used as a proxy for incidence/prevalence, these data can be useful. State health departments are also responsible for tracking notifiable diseases within their borders, relying on healthcare entities across the state to report these conditions. The reporting of notifiable conditions is fairly standardized and ultimately the CDC compiles data from the various states in a single database.

Beyond the reporting of mortality statistics and notifiable diseases, state health departments vary in the types of relevant data they collect and disseminate. Some states maintain registries of various health conditions with the intent of tracking cancer, heart disease, injuries, or some other indicator of morbidity. States typically participate in the Behavioral Risk Factor Surveillance Survey and may supplement the CDC questionnaire with customized survey items and/or expand the sampling frame in order to be able to examine health issues for sub-state geographical units.

The various states differ in the manner in which they maintain and disseminate data useful for morbidity analysis. Some states report data below the state level but virtually never below the county level. Thus, while analysis can be carried out at the county level in some cases, it is often impossible to access data for the level of analysis that may be desired. (A limitation affecting use of any health department-generated data is the almost fanatical concern over inadvertent disclosure of personal data.)

Depending on the organization of state government, state health departments may have responsibility for the administration of other functions that involve the generation of morbidity data. For example, some health departments manage the environmental protection agencies for their respective states (in addition to the routine environmental monitoring that is performed), and in this capacity collect data on health conditions resulting from environmental pollution.

Some state health departments are responsible for licensing and/or monitoring health facilities. In states that require hospitals to submit annual reports of their activities, the health department may be involved in compiling and analyzing data from these reports whether or not they are the administering agency. While these reports may be limited in detail related to morbidity, it may be possible to determine the types of cases that are being treated at the respective facilities. Thus, it is typical to solicit information on the number of patients that were seen in various specialties (e.g., OB-GYN, pediatrics, cardiology). Further, in states that require hospitals to submit utilization data, the health department may be responsible for managing that database.

In some states, the health department may have oversight of health insurance companies and/or manage the state Medicaid program. In these states, the department may collect data on medical claims from private and/or public insurance plans. Claims data are essentially utilization data and can be used to a certain extent as proxies for incidence/prevalence. In addition to routine monitoring of data in these domains, health departments may conduct special studies focusing on a particular health threat (e.g., domestic violence), a particular disease (e.g., HIV/AIDS), or a particular segment of the population (e.g., pregnant women).

Some of the functions described above may be assigned to a state agency other than the health department and these agencies, thus, become additional sources of morbidity data. Most states have an environmental protection agency of some type that may collect and disseminate data on pollution-related health conditions. In some states oversight of health insurance activities may be accorded to a specific agency. That agency may have oversight of Medicaid as well as private health insurance, although Medicaid may be assigned to a separate agency.

In recent years, several states have established databases that aggregate health insurance claims information from all healthcare payers into a statewide information repository. While these databases are designed to support cost containment and quality improvement efforts, the claims data (which include diagnosis) can serve as something of a proxy for morbidity data. Participating stakeholders may include private health insurers, Medicaid, children's health insurance and state employee health benefit programs, prescription drug plans, dental insurers, self-insured employer plans, and Medicare. The databases contain claims data (medical, pharmacy, and dental) and are used to report cost, use, and quality information. The data consist of "service-level" information based on valid claims processed by these healthcare payers. Service-level information includes among other variables clinical diagnosis, procedure codes, and patient demographics. To mask the identity of patients and ensure privacy, states usually encrypt, aggregate, and suppress patient identifiers. These databases are only available for certain states and the ability to access the data therein varies by state as well.

One other potential source of data at the state government level is public institutions of higher education. State-funded universities typically have numerous research institutes and a commitment to community service. They may be subcontracted by the state in fact to analyze if not manage health-related data. Many universities receive grant funds for purposes of studying morbidity patterns within the state's communities, with departments of public health and state-funded medical schools having a particular interest in the health status of the state's population.

Limited morbidity data is generated by local governments, although some larger cities may have departments that address factors related to health. The county health department is clearly a source of mortality data and certain morbidity data. Planning agencies, while typically not in the health data collection business, may compile health data from other sources for use, for example, in a health impact analysis.

This does not exhaust the list of government sources of data on morbidity but only provides a sampler. Publications of the federal National Technical Information Service (NTIS) provide a good starting point for finding other relevant databases.

Association Data Sources

The number and type of associations that are involved in collecting, analyzing, and/or disseminating morbidity data continues to grow. Some of these organizations are devoted to a particular disease (e.g., American Heart Association, Diabetes Foundation) or a particular segment of the population (e.g., March of Dimes). Others tend to represent professional interests and are typically not disease or population specific (e.g., National Association of Health Data Organizations, Academy Health). These organizations contribute to our understanding of morbidity patterns in a variety of ways. Some of them are involved in primary research (e.g., Planned Parenthood), compilation and analysis of data from other sources (e.g., American Cancer Society), or simply repackaging data from other sources (e.g., American Association of Retired People).

Whether the organization is involved primarily in data collection, data analysis, or data dissemination, these associations represent a significant source of data for those who do not have an in-depth understanding of data sources. Many of them publish "fact sheets" which for many can be the starting point for more in-depth research. Associations established to promote a particular health cause or to help fight a certain disease are likely to compile and disseminate data relevant to their areas of interest. Exhibit 9.5 presents an example of a statistical overview from the American Heart Association.

Exhibit 9.5: Stroke Statistics

The following is an excerpt from a "fact sheet" displayed online by the American Heart Association:

- In 2010, worldwide prevalence of stroke was 33 million, with 16.9 million people having a first stroke.
- Stroke was the second-leading global cause of death behind heart disease, accounting for 11.13 % of total deaths worldwide.
- Stroke is the number 5 cause of death in the United States, killing nearly 129000 people a year.
- Stroke kills someone in the US about once every 4 minutes.
- African-Americans have nearly twice the risk for a first-ever stroke than white people, and a much higher death rate from stroke.
- Over the past 10 years, the death rate from stroke has fallen about 35 % and the number of stroke deaths has dropped about 21 %.
- About 795000 people have a stroke every year.
- Someone in the US has a stroke about once every 40 seconds.
- Stroke causes 1 of every 20 deaths in the US.
- Stroke is a leading cause of disability.
- Stroke is the leading preventable cause of disability.

Source: American Heart Association. Retrieved from http://www.heart.org/idc/groups/ahamah-public/@wcm/@sop/@smd/documents/downloadable/ucm_470704.pdf

---

The American Public Health Association is an example of an "industry association" that among its many purposes is the dissemination of health data. "Public health data" could include about anything and the range of data of interest to public health officials and researchers is indeed broad. While the APHA does not conduct much primary research on morbidity, its member organizations and researchers do, making the organization an important channel for the distribution of such information.

Also included in the association category for our purposes are research institutes, many of which are affiliated with universities. Much like the associations referenced above, these research institutes may perform primary research, analyze their data or someone else's, or be primarily involved in the repackaging and dissemination of data from other sources. The Women's Health Research Institute at Northwestern

University, for example, offers a guide to data on sex differences in morbidity for various conditions. The Rand Corporation, although considered a private organization, is perhaps more akin to the research institutes noted here in terms of its commitment to advancing knowledge on health status.

Some organizations that are not generators of morbidity data themselves may be involved in encouraging, facilitating, or disseminating morbidity data on the part of others. The National Association of Health Data Organizations plays such a role and, while not in a position to provide data itself, may provide guidance in identifying other sources. Philanthropic foundations may also be involved in compiling, analyzing, and disseminating morbidity data. Some, like the Kaiser Family Foundation, may conduct primary research.

Hospital associations of various types may be involved in the compilation of data from participating hospitals. Increasingly, hospital associations have come to take a more active role in the activities of their member organizations, and the compilation, analysis and/or dissemination of data is an area where considerable activity has occurred. Most hospital associations are organized at the state level (since facilities are regulated at that level), and the role of the hospital association varies from state to state. In some cases, the associations themselves have established health data repositories, while in other cases state regulations that mandate the submission of hospital data to the state make the hospital association the logical "home" for such data. (In other cases, the state health department or some other agency may have this responsibility.) The primary benefit of these repositories from the perspective of morbidity analysis is the compilation of data on diagnosed conditions for hospital patients. Most of this information is restricted to inpatient care although a few states may collect data on hospital outpatient utilization (e.g., emergency department, surgery center, diagnostic center).

These data, of course, represent "known cases" and do not represent the totality of morbidity for any population or geographic area. Nevertheless, in the absence of any other source of information, data generated via these hospital association repositories represent a useful resource. It should be noted that access to the data generated via these association-managed databases varies from state to state; in some cases, a fee (sometimes substantial) may be charged for access and in others access may be limited to member organizations. Thus, the usefulness of these data sets will vary from state to state.

There has been a trend in recent years toward the establishment of regional health information organizations (RHIOs). Usually established as independent not-for-profit organizations, RHIOs are multi-stakeholder organizations created to facilitate the exchange of health information through the electronic transfer of health data among the stakeholders of that region's healthcare system. While primarily designed to improve the safety, quality, and efficiency of healthcare, RHIOs may also support research on the clinical data accumulated. RHIO stakeholders may include clinics, hospitals, medical societies, major employers, and insurers. The development of RHIOs nationwide has been uneven and the number of successful ventures is not large at this point. RHIOs typically start by collecting hospital data some of which can be used as a proxy for morbidity. A small number compile data on ambulatory services from physician offices and clinics. These offer insights into the health conditions for those presenting to physician offices. Even access to this scant information is limited in that RHIOs typically have strict rules regarding access to the data—in most cases, limited to the participating stakeholders.

Commercial Data Sources

As the demand for health data has grown, a number of commercial operations have been established to generate various types of data while other, existing organizations have added health data to their offerings. Since there is no central repository for morbidity data, these organizations face the same limitations that other data generators face, and some of them serve the same purposes as entities noted above under the governmental and association sections.

Some commercial operations compile hospital utilization data and more than one has attempted to develop a nationwide database. Others have compiled insurance claims data and, similarly, attempted to create a national database. None of these efforts to develop a universal set of data have been very successful. These entities are primarily collecting utilization data (either directly from healthcare providers or from the insurance companies that process the claims). Some examples of these organizations are Truven Health and IMS Health. However obtained, these data involve "known cases" and can serve as only a proxy for morbidity data. Some data vendors extract data from government surveys (e.g., from NCHS and the CDC) and repackage the information for their clients. A few companies conduct national health surveys or broad consumer surveys that include a health component. Simmons Consumer Research annually surveys 25000 households and collects, among other information, data on the presence of a wide range of health conditions. IMS Health is the primary aggregator of drug prescription data, and this information (which must be purchased) is thought to serve as a proxy for disease incidence/prevalence (Cossman et al. 2010).

Synthetic Data

Synthetic data have long been used by demographers in the absence of actual data, with synthetic data increasingly being generated to estimate the level of morbidity within a population. Synthetic data are created by merging existing demographic data with observed rates of disease incidence/prevalence and/or service utilization to produce estimates, projections, and forecasts.

The general approach involves applying known rates for a defined population to a current or projected population figure. To the extent possible, these rates are adjusted for, at a minimum, the age and sex composition of the targeted population. Rates for the incidence/prevalence of various health conditions and for the utilization of health services generated by the National Center for Health Statistics are the basis for most such calculations. The demographic data may be obtained from a variety of sources.

Exhibit 9.6 provides a simple example of the generation of prevalence rates for asthma for a defined population. As if often the case, rates for males and females are calculated separately and then combined, since the observed risk of morbidity for virtually every conditions varies by sex.

Exhibit 9.6: Calculating Prevalence Rates

The following table illustrates the process used to synthetically generate a prevalence rate.

Age cohort	Prevalence Estimate			Prevalence Estimate		
	Males	Rate/1000	Cases	Females	Rate/1000	Cases
0–14	1000	100	100	1000	80	80
15–24	1000	70	70	1000	60	60
25–44	2000	40	80	2200	30	66
45–64	1500	20	30	1800	15	27
65+500	10	5	800	5	4	
Total	6000		285	6800		237

The population in each cohort is multiplied by the rate for that age group to generate the estimated number of cases for the year in question. The cases generated for each cohort of males and females are summed to yield the total number of cases for males and the total number of cases for females. These two figures are subsequently combined to generate the total estimated prevalence. For this population of 12800 with this age/sex distribution, an estimate of 522 cases of asthma is generated for the current year. This yields an incidence rate of 40 cases per 1000 persons.

The demand for synthetic data is being met by both government agencies and commercial data vendors. However, government agencies seldom provide the synthetic data in the format needed, and commercial vendors and consultants represent a more ready source if any level of granularity is required. Some vendors such as Health and Performance Resources have developed calculations for the full range of diseases as well as demand estimates for various services. Other vendors may specialize in data, for example, on a particular health condition or the demand for a particular service line. Typically, these data are not in the public domain but available only to customers of the vendors.

Estimates and projections of morbidity have become essential for virtually any planning, marketing, or business development activity in healthcare, and there has been growing pressure for the generation of increasingly detailed figures. However, there are at least three major concerns related to the use of such data. First, the estimates and projections are based on historical prevalence rates at a time when patterns of morbidity are undergoing change. Second, the results of such calculations may vary depending on the source of demographic data. Third, estimates and projections become increasingly tenuous as the size of the geography becomes smaller. While synthetic morbidity rates may be fairly dependable down to even the county level, they tend to become unstable when sub-county units such as zip codes or census tracts are considered. Despite these caveats, the demand for estimates and projections of morbidity will continue to grow as long as there is interest in the current and future level of morbidity within the US population.

Assessment of Data Options

Having reviewed the sources of morbidity data available on the US population, it might be useful to assess the options that are available in terms of their usefulness to applied demographers. In terms of the overall availability of morbidity data it must be conceded that, relative to fertility and mortality data, the options are limited. The primary generators of morbidity data (i.e., federal agencies like the CDC and NCHS) do compile significant amounts of data through registries and surveys. The most comprehensive compilation of such data is represented by the annual reports of notifiable diseases from the Centers for Disease Control and Prevention. However, this information is limited to communicable diseases and, as such, omits the types of conditions that are responsible for 95 % of the population's morbidity today.

The surveys conducted by the CDC, NCHS, and other federal agencies do generate morbidity data but with important limitations. Community-based surveys (such as the NCHS National Health Interview Survey) collect a limited amount of morbidity data through self-reports and on-site examinations, and the CDC's BRFSS collects data from a sample of the population on diagnoses they have received and on their use of services for selected health problems. The data generated are based primarily on self-reports with all the caveats that implies and, in any case, such surveys can only deal with a relative handful of the thousands of health conditions that could affect the population.

To the extent that these data are compiled and disseminated, they have clear limitations for those who want to apply them to concrete situations. The time period between data collection and the publication of results may be lengthy, several years in some cases, although some CDC and NCHS reports are produced in an expeditious manner. More important, however, is the geographic granularity of the data. Data on notifiable diseases, for example, are only available at the state level. This is not very useful for most analyses and, although point data is available to the CDC, data confidentiality rules restrict access for most analysts to this granular data. BRFSS data are primarily published at the state level, with some data available at the county level. However, for most counties the sample size is too small to be meaningful (except in cases where an individual county has paid to expand the sample size).

The most useful sources of detailed morbidity data for most purposes are generated by NCHS surveys. The NHIS mentioned above generates some data on morbidity, although the small number of conditions it tracks changes over time. The surveys of hospital data and physician office data yield detailed data on the types of conditions for which people are admitted to hospitals and the conditions for which people seek physician services. While a wealth of information is generated these data represent known cases and do not necessarily reflect the true level of disease within the population. Even more important, the rates that these surveys yield are typically not available for populations below the regional level. Thus, for most applications, national incidence and prevalence rates must be applied to local populations, regardless of how the local population differs from the national population in terms of its demographic makeup.

The challenges involved in acquiring and using morbidity data were recently illustrated through a project carried out by the author (Thomas 2014). The project attempted to measure the extent to which contemporary Americans were actually getting sicker after decades of continuous health status improvement. In the absence of any central repository of morbidity data, it was necessary to acquire data from a variety of sources for specific conditions, with the various sources often covering different time periods and populations, and different methods of data collection. Many otherwise useful sources of data may have changed their definitions for certain conditions over time or discontinued data collection on certain conditions at a point in time. The analysis involved putting together a "patchwork quilt" of data and noting the numerous caveats that had to be considered. Although there was the occasional aggregate measure (e.g., "chronic disease") that could be tracked, even there the data trail did not extend very far back into the past. At the end of the day, it was not possible to conclude based on the data that could be compiled on whether Americans are getting sicker or not. The best that could be done was to track changes in Condition A, Condition B, or Condition C and draw conclusions based on fragmented data.

As noted above, certain associations and private data vendors have attempted to make more morbidity data available to the public. However, to the extent that most of this involves the repackaging of government data, researchers who are familiar with the original sources are not likely to benefit. The most useful benefit provided by commercial data vendors is represented by their efforts to generate synthetic data in the form of estimates and projections of the incidence/prevalence of various conditions and the use of various health services. Because data generation is based on rates, it is possible to generate estimates/projections for virtually any geographic area or subpopulation (assuming that the requisite demographic data are available). Despite the tremendous potential here for acquiring detailed data for virtually any defined population, this information is considered proprietary and is made available only to customers of the data vendors. Anyone can become a customer, of course, but this often involves a significant investment. At the time of this writing, another consideration is that NCHS has not released national and regional rates for these models since 2010. Thus, estimates and projections made available today may reflect rates of morbidity and/or health status that are no longer valid.

The inadequacy of morbidity data is a problem that everyone recognizes but no party is in a position to effect much meaningful change. Federal agencies have a commitment to make as much useful data available as possible but are chronically limited due to funding shortfalls. Commercial data vendors are limited in their data generation due to the lag in the generation of rates by federal agencies. For the present, researchers and analysts must be content with a situation in which there are significant limitations on the ability to conduct research on the level of morbidity of the US population.

References

Cossman, R. E., James, W. L., Cossman, J. S., et al. (2010, March). Prescription data as a proxy for disease prevalence in the Mississippi delta. *ResearchGate.* Retrieved from http://www.researchgate.net/publication/252931404_Prescription_Data_as_a_Proxy_for_County_Level_Illness_Prevalence_in_the_Mississippi_Delta.

Thomas, R. K. (2014, January 12). Are Americans getting sicker: emerging morbidity trends. Presented at the bi-annual meeting of the Applied Demography Conference, San Antonio, TX.

Additional Resources

American Public Health Association (www.apha).
Centers for Disease Control and Prevention (www.cdc.gov).
Health & Performance Resources (www.hpranalytics.com).
Kaiser Family Foundation (www.kff.org).
National Association of Health Data Organizations (www.nahdo.org).
National Center for Health Statistics (www.cdc.gov/nchs).
National Institutes of Health (www.nih.gov).
Rand Center for Population Health and Health Disparities (www.rand.org).
Women's Health Research Institute at Northwestern University (https://www.womenshealth.northwestern.edu/about-institute).

Glossary

Acquired immunodeficiency syndrome (AIDS)   Immune deficiency caused by human immunodeficiency virus (HIV).

Activities of daily living (ADLs)   Activities related to personal care that include bathing or showering, dressing, getting into or out of bed or a chair, using the toilet, and eating.

Admission, hospital   Any person, excluding newborns, accepted for inpatient services during the survey reporting period.

Age adjustment   A statistical adjustment used to compare risks for two or more populations at one point in time or for one population at two or more points in time. Age-adjusted rates are computed by the direct method by applying age-specific rates in a population of interest to a standardized age distribution, to eliminate differences in observed rates that result from age differences in population composition.

Average length of stay   Average length of stay in a hospital is computed by dividing the total number of hospital days of care (counting the date of admission but not the date of discharge) by the number of patients discharged. The American Hospital Association computes average length of stay by dividing the number of inpatient days by the number of admissions.

Basic actions difficulty   Limitations or difficulties in movement, emotional, sensory, or cognitive functioning associated with a health problem.

Birth weight   The first weight of the newborn obtained after birth. Low birth weight is defined as weighing less than 2500 g (5 lb 8 oz). Very low birth weight is defined as weighing less than 1500 g (3 lb 4 oz).

Blood pressure, high   An average systolic blood pressure reading of at least 140 mmHg or diastolic reading of at least 90 mmHgn.

Body mass index (BMI)   A measure calculated as weight divided by height. Healthy weight for adults is defined as a BMI of 18.5 to less than 25; overweight

© Springer New York 2016
R.K. Thomas, *In Sickness and In Health*, Applied Demography Series 6,
DOI 10.1007/978-1-4939-3423-2

(including obese), as a BMI greater than or equal to 25; and obesity, as a BMI greater than or equal to 30.

Cause of death   The underlying medical condition reported on the death certificate that resulted in the death of the individual.

Cholesterol   The combination of high-density lipoproteins (HDLs), low-density lipoproteins (LDLs), and very-low-density lipoproteins (VLDLs) determined through a blood test. High serum total cholesterol is a risk factor for cardiovascular disease.

Complex activity limitation   A measure of disability defined by the inability to function successfully in certain social roles. Complex activities consist of the tasks and organized activity that make up numerous social roles like working, maintaining a household, living independently, or participating in community activities.

Condition, health   A departure from a state of physical or mental well-being.

Days of care   The number of adult and pediatric days of hospital care rendered during the entire reporting period. Days of care for newborns are excluded.

Dental caries   Evidence of dental decay on any surface of a tooth.

Diabetes   A group of conditions in which insulin is not adequately secreted or utilized. Diabetes is a leading cause of disease and death in the United States.

Discharge, hospital   Release from a hospital or other medical facility at the completion of any continuous period of stay of one night or more as an inpatient.

Emergency department or emergency room visit   Any visit to a hospital emergency department for the purpose of seeking care and receiving personal health services for an immediate problem.

End-stage renal disease (ESRD)   The complete or near complete failure of the kidneys to function to excrete wastes, concentrate urine, and regulate electrolytes. ESRD occurs when the kidneys are no longer able to function at the level necessary for day-to-day life.

Gestation   The period beginning with the first day of the last normal menstrual period and ending with the day of birth or day of termination of pregnancy.

Health status, respondent-assessed   A state of health determined by asking the respondent about whether his or her health is excellent, very good, good, fair, or poor?" The health status of a group may be computed by aggregating responses for individuals.

Hospital utilization   Estimates of hospital utilization include hospital discharge rate, days of care rate, average length of stay, and percentage of the population with a hospitalization.

Human immunodeficiency virus (HIV) disease   A disease caused by infection with a cytopathic retrovirus, which in turn leads to destruction of parts of the immune system.

Incidence   The number of cases of disease having occurred during a prescribed period of time. It is often expressed as a rate (e.g., the incidence of measles per 1000 children 5–15 years of age during a specified year).

Injury   A (suspected) bodily lesion resulting from acute overexposure to energy (this can be mechanical, thermal, electrical, chemical, or radiant) interacting with the body in amounts or rates that exceed the threshold of physiological tolerance.

Injury-related visit   An emergency department visit is considered injury-related if the physician's diagnosis was injury-related (*International Classification of Diseases, 9th Revision, Clinical Modification* (ICD–9–CM, code 800–999)), an external cause-of-injury code was present (ICD–9–CME800–E999), or the patient's reason for visit code was injury-related.

Inpatient   Any person who is formally admitted to the inpatient service of a hospital for observation, care, diagnosis, or treatment.

Instrumental activities of daily living (IADLs)   Activities related to independent living that include preparing meals, managing money, shopping for groceries or personal items, performing light or heavy housework, and using a telephone.

International Classification of Diseases (ICD)   A disease classification system developed collaboratively by the World Health Organization and ten international centers to promote international comparability in the collection, classification, processing, and presentation of health statistics.

Life expectancy   The average number of years of life remaining to a person at a particular age based on a given set of age-specific death rates.

Limitation of activity   A long-term reduction in a person's capacity to perform the usual kind or amount of activities associated with his or her age group as a result of a chronic condition.

Long-term care facility   A residence that provides a specified level of personal or medical care or supervision to residents for an extended period of time.

Mammography   A type of imaging that generates an X-ray image of the breast used to detect irregularities in breast tissue.

Mental health organization   An administratively distinct public or private agency or institution whose primary concern is provision of direct mental health services to the mentally ill or emotionally disturbed.

Notifiable disease   A condition that healthcare providers are required, usually by law, to report to state or local public health officials. Notifiable diseases are those of public interest by reason of their contagiousness, severity, or frequency.

Nursing home   A facility that provides long-term custodial care for dependent patients.

Office visit   Any visit to a physician's ambulatory practice (office) location other than in a hospital, nursing home, other extended care facility, patient's home, industrial clinic, college clinic, or family planning clinic.

Outpatient department   A hospital facility where non-urgent ambulatory medical care is provided.

Outpatient visit   A visit for receipt of medical, dental, or other services at a hospital by patients who are not admitted to the hospital.

Outpatient surgery   A surgical operation, whether major or minor, performed on patients who do not remain in the hospital overnight.

Prenatal care   Medical care provided to a pregnant woman to prevent complications and decrease the incidence of maternal and prenatal mortality.

Prevalence   The number of cases of a disease, number of infected persons, or number of persons with some other attribute present during a particular interval of time. It is often expressed as a rate (e.g., the prevalence of diabetes per 1000 persons during a year).

Rate   A measure of some event, disease, or condition in relation to a unit of population, along with some specification of time.

Serious psychological distress   A measure of psychological distress associated with unspecified but potentially diagnosable mental illness that may result in a higher risk for disability and higher utilization of health services.

Substance use   Substance use refers to the use of selected substances, including alcohol, tobacco products, drugs, inhalants, and other substances that can be consumed, inhaled, injected, or otherwise absorbed into the body with possible dependence and other detrimental effects.

Usual source of care   Access to a physician, clinic or other healthcare provider ususally for primary care.

Index

© Springer New York 2016
R.K. Thomas, *In Sickness and In Health*, Applied Demography Series 6,
DOI 10.1007/978-1-4939-3423-2